Training Guide To Cerebral Palsy Sports

The Recognized Training Guide of the
United States Cerebral Palsy Athletic Association

Third Edition

Jeffery A. Jones, MPE
Editor

Human Kinetics Books
Champaign, Illinois

Library of Congress Cataloging-in-Publication Data
Training guide to cerebral palsy sports.

  Bibliography: p.
  1. Sports for the handicapped—United States.
2. Cerebral palsy. I. Jones, Jeffery A., 1956-
II. United States Cerebral Palsy Athletic Association.
GV709.3.T73   1988   796'.01'96   87-3081
ISBN 0-87322-125-7

Developmental Editor: Jan Progen, EdD
Production Director: Ernie Noa
Projects Manager: Lezli Harris
Assistant Editor: Phaedra A. Hise
Copy Editor: Ann Bruehler
Typesetter: Sonnie Bowman
Proofreader: Laurie McGee
Text Layout: Cathy Romans
Text Design: Keith Blomberg
Illustrator: Marvin Teeples
Cover Design: Conundrum Designs
Printed By: Versa Press

ISBN: 0-87322-125-7

Printed in the United States of America

10 9 8 7 6 5 4 3 2 1

Human Kinetics Books
A Division of Human Kinetics Publishers, Inc.
Box 5076, Champaign, IL 61820
1-800-DIAL-HKP
1-800-334-3665 (in Illinois)

To Kristyn Andrea Jones
Love
Dad

Contents

Preface

This manual represents the efforts and experiences of more than 40 individuals throughout the country. The articles not only cover the different sports offered by the United States Cerebral Palsy Athletic Association, they also include a variety of topics ranging from flexibility and endurance training to an adaptive aerobics program. As you read through the chapters, you will find some of them are very specific to cerebral palsy (CP) sports, whereas others rarely even use the words physical disability. This illustrates that the essence of CP sports is just that: *sports*.

Many of the same coaching strategies and training techniques applicable for able-bodied athletes are described with respect to athletes with CP and other physical disabilities. The athletes discussed within this manual are athletes first and individuals with CP second. This manual should clearly illustrate that the only difference between a CP athlete and his or her able-bodied counterpart is that CP athletes have a few extra obstacles to deal with before crossing the finish line. The most obvious, of course, are the physical obstacles of their disabilities. However, athletes with physical disabilities often have to cope with inaccessible facilities, lack of competitive opportunities, limited budgets, and ignorance on the part of service providers, facility operators, and sports and recreation professionals.

Fortunately, these obstacles are slowly disappearing. Since the establishment of the Committee on Sports for the Disabled (an official subcommittee of the United States Olympic Committee), great strides have been accomplished. Demonstration events involving physically disabled athletes were held as part of the 1984 Summer and Winter Olympics and have since become a regular part of the annual United States Olympic Festival, as well as part of the 1986 U.S. Outdoor Track and Field championships.

This continued acceptance by the able-bodied sports community is due in part to a transformation of the disabled sports movement from being mainly a recreationally based program to being a wide spectrum of competitive sports opportunities for well-trained, well-coached athletes. This transition has been very apparent in the CP sports movement. The past 3 years have seen the formation of the American Cerebral Palsy/Les Autres Coaches Association and a complete restructuring of its national sports office. We are a part of a young and ever growing sports organization. Continued research, ongoing cooperation with other sports organizations (serving both disabled and able-bodied athletes), and a higher quality of athletic competition are all part of the future of the United States Cerebral Palsy Athletic Association.

This manual suggests that another part of that future includes the continued development of coaching expertise. It takes more than sports knowledge to be successful in the area of sports for athletes with physical disabilities. As many of the enclosed articles will indicate, coaches need both creativity and enthusiasm in order to be successful. CP sports continually present an array of challenging opportunities to both coaches and athletes. This third edition of the *Training Guide to Cerebral Sports* outlines many of these opportunities and invites the reader to participate. Be a part of the excitement!

Acknowledgments

Besides the thousands of athletes and coaches across the country who collectively make cerebral palsy sports what they are today, and the host of coaches, educators, and sport practitioners who have contributed their expertise to this manual, I would like to thank a number of key individuals and organizations for their involvement in this project.

First, I thank the Board of Directors of both the United States Cerebral Palsy Athletic Association and the Michigan Cerebral Palsy/Les Autres Sports Association for their assistance and support. Their insight and direction regarding sport opportunities for individuals with cerebral palsy helped to establish the parameters from which this manual was developed. My sincere appreciation is also extended to the officers and members of the American Cerebral Palsy/Les Autres Coaches Association for their continued efforts in the promotion of CP/LA Sports.

Acknowledgments are also extended to Trudy Budziak, Margaret Johnson, and Dorothy McClure for their clerical and editorial assistance, as well as Marvin Teeples, the creative illustrator, whose talent is demonstrated throughout these pages. I also thank Peter Gregson, my wife MaryBeth Jones, and Elizabeth Palnick for providing the photographs and slides on which most of the illustrations were based.

Finally, I would like to thank Claudine Sherrill for her support and initial introduction to Human Kinetics Publishers, for without that informal introduction and the tremendous support and assistance of Rainer Martens and Human Kinetics Publishers, this manual would have been impossible.

Acknowledgment

Contributors

Bob Accorsi
  Recreation and Leisure Services
  Springfield College
  Springfield, MA 01109

Libby Anderson
  1435 33rd Street
  San Diego, CA 92102

Robert Bergquist, MPE, RPT
  Associate Professor
  HPERPT Division
  Springfield College
  Springfield, MA 01108

Natalie Bieber
  Town Woods Road
  Lyme, CT 06371

Raphael Bieber
  640 Ditmas Avenue
  Brooklyn, NY 11218

F.R.S. Binding, PhD
  Social Psychologist
  300 Regina N #1–206
  Waterloo, Ontario N2J 3138

George S. Brown
  326 North Quaker Lane
  West Hartford, CT 06119

F. John Bugbee
  Springfield Technical
    Community College
  Springfield, MA 01108

Ruth Burd
  Team Services
    Physical Therapist
  2901 LaVista Court
  Decatur, GA 30033

Barbara Cancilla
  Director of Avon Physical
    Therapy Association
  54 W. Avon Road
  Avon, CT 06001

Scott Cusimano
  220 G. South West
  Ardmore, OK 73401

Gerry Dausman
  Program Developer
  National Rifle Association
  1600 Rhode Island Avenue, N.W.
  Washington, DC 20036

Ronald Davis, PhD
  Ball State University
    Special Physical Education
  Muncie, IN 47306

Kim Grass
  DeKalb County School System
  2112 Seaman Circle
  Atlanta, GA 30341

Jeffery A. Jones
  Sports and Recreation Consultant
  31505 Kathryn
  Garden City, MI 48135

MaryBeth Jones
  Therapeutic Recreation Consultant
  31505 Kathryn
  Garden City, MI 48135

Fred Koch
  Director of Physical Education
    UCP of New York City
  175 Lawrence Avenue
  Brooklyn, NY 11230

Jerry Lewis
  70 Washington Avenue
  Iselin, NJ 08830

Jamy Black McCole
  1932 6th Avenue
  Fort Worth, TX 76110

Jerry McCole, Director
  Dallas Riders Disabled
    Sports Association
  P.O. Box 3044
  Dallas, TX 75221-3044

Alfred Morris, PhD, FACSM
Armed Forces Staff College
7800 Hampton Boulevard
Norfolk, VA 23511

Carol Mushett
Recreational Therapist
Sinai Hospital of Detroit
6767 West Outer Drive
Detroit, MI 48235

Michael P. Mushett
Sports & Recreation Consultant
34299 Claudia Court
Westland, MI 48185

James Patterson
Development Office
University of Texas
200 West 21st Street
Austin, TX 78712

Grant Peacock, MED, RPT
Peacock Physical Therapy, Inc.
3132 Bomar Forest Place
Decatur, GA 30033

Marilyn Pink
Director of Biomechanics
Centinela Hospital
555 E. Hardy Street
P.O. Box 720
Inglewood, CA 90307

Pat Pride
Recreation Therapy Supervisor
Magee Rehabilitation Hospital
6 Franklin Plaza
Philadelphia, PA 19106

Phil Roberts
34 French Street
Bristol, CT 06010

Paul Roper
Southern Connecticut State
University
New Haven, CT 06515

Karen Rusling, RPT
495 Rainbow Road
Windsor, CT 06095

Gregory B. Shasby, PhD
Assistant Professor of
Physical Education
University of Virginia
Charlottesville, VA 22903

Claudine Sherrill
Texas Women's University
P.O. Box 23717
Denton, TX 76204

Dave Stephenson
1101 Post Oak Boulevard
Houston, TX 77056

Janice Tetreault
5 Beachwood Drive
North Kingstown, RI 02852

Paul Tetreault
5 Beachwood Drive
North Kingstown, RI 02852

Part I

Introduction to Cerebral Palsy Sports

Sports Opportunities for Individuals With Cerebral Palsy: A Brief Historical Perspective

Jeffery A. Jones

For many years individuals with cerebral palsy (CP) have been told by parents, educators, and physicians that sports were something to watch from a distance, never something to participate in. The more physically involved the individual was, the more ridiculous was the thought of actually participating in competitive sports. Fortunately, through the efforts of a constantly growing number of dedicated individuals and the United States Cerebral Palsy Athletic Association (USCPAA), hundreds of local programs across the country have been making exception to that myth for the past 10 years. Sports are certainly not for everyone. However, the 780 athletes who competed in the Fifth National Cerebral Palsy Games and the thousands of other CP athletes across the country are showing parents, educators, and physicians that individuals with CP can be and are *athletes*.

The Beginning

The first organized, nationwide sports program specifically serving the athletic needs of individuals with CP began in 1978 with the establishment of the National Association of Sports for Cerebral Palsy (NASCP). It was determined that at that point in the development of sports opportunities for individuals with disabilities within the United States, the existing groups could not appropriately meet the needs of the CP athlete.

After hosting its first national competition in Detroit, Michigan, in 1978, NASCP began to encourage the development of local teams who trained in community-based recreation facilities, schools, hospitals, nonprofit organizations such as United Cerebral Palsy Associations and Easter Seal Society, and independent sports clubs. NASCP helped organize and sponsor local, state, and regional competitions yearly and National Games biannually. Outstanding athletes were selected to United States teams according to their performances at National Games. International competitions are held on even-numbered years and are sponsored by Cerebral Palsy–International Sports and Recreation Association (CP-ISRA).

Shortly after the 1979 National Games, NASCP became a program of United Cerebral Palsy Associations (UCPA), Inc., and a Group E member of the United States Olympic Committee, specifically, the Committee on Sports for the Disabled (COSD). Both events proceeded to have significant impact on the future development of CP sports.

Program Component of UCPA

Affiliation with UCPA established NASCP as a program component under the direction of the Consumer Activities Department. NASCP and the nationwide program it represented developed tremendously through this newly established affiliation. The quality of coaching as well as the quality of athletic competition steadily improved. Simultaneously, NASCP experienced a significant increase in participation. Numbers of athletes at national competitions grew from 128 in 1978 to 780 in 1985, even with the use of a third consecutive increase in qualifying standards. Table 1 lists the years the Games were held, the host states, and the number of competitors for each of the past five National Games.

Program increase was also measured by the number of participating athletes. As of the spring, 1986, approximately 3,000 athletes from more than 125 individual sports teams in 38 states were participating in more than 60 local, state, and regional competitions nationwide.

Time for Transition

After more than 5 years of extensive program development under the auspices of UCPA, a movement began early in 1985 to restructure the administrative component of NASCP. A large portion of NASCP membership believed it was time for the association to be represented by an independent national governing body (NGB) similar in structure and function to that of the other NGBs. At that time, NASCP was the only sports organization not independently running its national program.

After nearly 16 months of negotiations, the transition was made official with the first Board of Directors meeting of the newly formed, independent NGB. As of November 1986, NASCP would be known as the United States Cerebral Palsy Athletic Association (USCPAA). The only major difference in program operations is that now USCPAA is represented by its own Board of Directors and subcommittee structure, functioning independently from the day-to-day policy decisions of UCPA.

Table 1   Year, Location, and Number of Participating Athletes in the National Cerebral Palsy Games.

Year	Location	Number of competitors
1978	Detroit, MI	128
1979	New Haven, CT	321
1981	Kingston, RI	450
1983	Ft. Worth, TX	753
1985	East Lansing, MI	780

The significance of this transition is primarily focused on the future growth potential of USCPAA. Under the program structure of NASCP/UCPA, program growth was substantial for the first 5 years. Then growth began to stagnate because of UCPA's priority to its affiliates. This stagnation was understandable because that priority is one of the primary mission statements of National UCPA. The change to an independent NGB now allows an across-the-board emphasis on program development. School-based programs, community park and recreation departments, hospitals, independent sports programs, and UCPA-affiliated programs will all be treated with the same priority.

USOC: Group E Member

USCPAA is much more than a single organization working for the development of CP sports. USCPAA is an intricate part of a national and international network of sports organizations. Nationally, USCPAA is one of seven member groups represented on the COSD, a recognized subcommittee of the United States Olympic Committee.

Figure 1 depicts USCPAA's relationship to these various organizations. One reason for involvement is to assist in the continuing overall advancement of sports opportunities for all individuals with disabilities, regardless of the degree or nature of the disability. Through the combined efforts of all concerned, each organization (including USCPAA) will find the strength to grow and develop its own individual identity. Cooperation allows the opportunity to share ideas, learn from one another's mistakes and accomplishments, and solve common problems.

This sense of cooperation was evident in the recent formation of the United States Organization of Disabled Athletes (USODA). Established specifically for the promotion and development of four sports organizations (the United States Association for Blind Athletes, the United States Amputee Athletic Association, the United States Cerebral Palsy Athletic Association, and the Dwarf Athletic Association of America), USODA's goals are to provide a unique joint approach to fundraising, public relations, program promotion, and competition organization.

The seven organizations of COSD are not the only groups involved in the advancement of sports and recreation for individuals with disabilities. They are, however, the only ones funded in part by the United States Olympic Committee. A more extensive list of sports organizations can be found in Appendix A.

International Competition

The United States first began sending CP athletes to international competition in 1978 when 17 athletes attended the World CP Games in Edinborough, Scotland. That number grew to 49 in 1980 and 59 in 1982 when the United States team captured the world title at the Fifth International Cerebral Palsy Games in Greve, Denmark.

In 1984 the United States CP team joined forces with a unified United States contingent, including athletes from the United States Association for Blind Athletes (USABA), the United States Amputee Athletic Association (USAAA), and

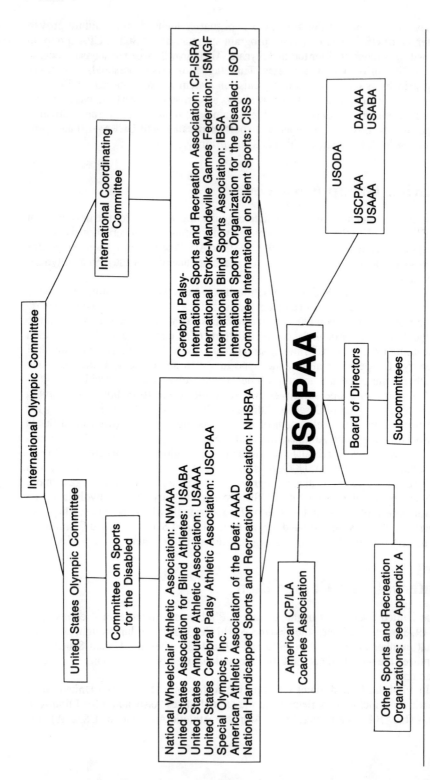

Figure 1. The USCPAA's relationship to the IOC and related organizations.

several "Les Autres" athletes, to participate in the 1984 International Games for The Disabled, a joint disability event held in Nassau County, New York and attracting more than 1,800 athletes from 41 countries around the world. Although the United States CP team lost a close medal count to Great Britain, the combined U.S. squad did capture first place in the overall medals count.

Concerns for the safety of travel in Europe was a contributing factor in the decision to withdraw the U.S. team from the 1986 International CP Games in Gits, Belgium. Approximately 30 of the 54 athletes selected to the 1986 U.S. Team traveled to Windsor, Canada in July 1986 to participate in an annual provisional Games as a substitute for the cancelled Belgium trip. Future international games are scheduled for Seoul, South Korea in 1988 and Holland in 1990.

Outside of team participation, CP athletes have represented the United States in international competition on several occasions. In 1980 a six-member equestrian team competed in Toronto, Canada. Later, in 1981, a Michigan contingent of four athletes and one coach traveled to Japan to participate in the Japanese National Games for The Disabled. Also in 1981, Sal Ficara, a Class VI athlete/coach from Hartford, Connecticut, was selected to participate in the Third International Disabled Games held in Rome.

The growth of CP sports in both the United States and Canada has also led to numerous joint competitions held in both the United States and neighboring Canada.

Les Autres: The Other Part of CP Sports

Although USCPAA is the governing body for sports competition for individuals with CP, it has in the past opened its doors to individuals with other developmental disabilities (such as multiple sclerosis, muscular dystrophy, arthrogryposis, and osteogenesis imperfecta) who were not presently being served by any other sport organization. Similar to their CP counterparts, these groups of Les Autres (French meaning, "The Others") athletes participate in local, regional, and national competition. An emphasis on the specific needs of Les Autres athletes began after the 1983 National Games when 72 Les Autres athletes participated on an integrated basis with the CP athletes. A more detailed discussion of Les Autres can be found in a subsequent section of this manual.

American CP/LA Coaches Association

Just recently, a group of sports practitioners organized and incorporated the American Cerebral Palsy/Les Autres Coaches Association, an organization devoted to the ongoing development of education and training opportunities for coaches working with physically disabled athletes.

Goals of the newly formed organization include

- providing expertise to such groups as community service centers, coaches of CP/LA athletes, university staff and students in disabled sports fields, community action groups, and so forth;

- disseminating information to any interested groups or individuals through materials such as newsletters, periodicals, monographs, pamphlets, news releases, and so forth;
- assisting in research studies designed to upgrade the understanding of problems involved in CP/LA sports and to upgrade the quality of coaching for disabled athletes;
- offering a forum through a newsletter *(The Mentor)* and other publications for CP/LA coaches to express views and gain insights in their work;
- forming a corps of coaches that will provide solidarity to the efforts of the CP/LA sports movement; and
- taking up any other cause that may serve the coaching and performance of CP/LA athletes.

Conclusion

What the future will bring to the development of CP sports in the United States is unclear. The very recent restructuring of the national organizations has established a very lengthy agenda. Possible priorities may include youth sports, the classification system, uniformity in games administration, certification of officials, and program development. What is clear is that the involvement of athletes, coaches, sports practitioners, and other interested individuals will certainly determine exactly what USCPAA's future agenda will be. Those presently involved understand that what makes sports so important to the individual with a disability is the total experience through participation. The process of learning how to win and lose, improving their functional abilities in an enjoyable atmosphere, developing greater ego strengths, and extending social and recreational experiences through participation in athletic competition is what is important. More important is the fact that CP sports are not services, but opportunities to work for a goal.

For more information on how you can be a part of this exciting sports movement and for more information about the CP sports team nearest you, contact one of the USCPAA representatives listed in Appendix B.

Note

For more information, contact: Rick Lander, 5805 Woodward, Merriman, KS 66202.

Cerebral Palsy and the CP Athlete

Claudine Sherrill
Carol Mushett
Jeffery A. Jones

Cerebral palsy (CP) is a group of neuromuscular conditions, not a disease. It is caused by damage to an area or areas of the brain that control and coordinate muscle tone, reflexes, and action. This brain damage can vary widely; therefore, the degree of muscular involvement in CP can range from severe spasticity to slight speech impairment. CP is not hereditary, contagious, or progressive (Jones, 1984).

The primary causes of CP take place during one of three stages of birth: (a) prenatally (prematurity, certain blood incompatibilities, and maternal illness); (b) natally (anoxia, trauma, and in the past, use of forceps); and (c) postnatally (infections, poisoning, trauma, and malnutrition).

Medical Versus Functional Classification

Types of CP are usually described medically two ways: type of muscular involvement and/or by areas in which the body is affected. Definitions of CP classified into the muscle involvement group include the following:

- *Spastic*—70% of cerebral palsied individuals are spastic, which is a constant state of hypertonus, usually involving flexor muscle groups. This condition is due to exaggerated reflex levels normally under voluntary control. Cortical level damage is implied here, which is the highest level of control.
- *Athetoid*—20 to 30% of cerebral palsied individuals have athetoid involvement, implying basal ganglia damage, resulting in slow, writhing, vermicular type movements that may affect the trunk and proximal extremities (dystonic) and abrupt jerky distal movements (choreiform). Often these movements increase with emotion and stress. Dysarthria is often attached to this involvement.
- *Ataxia*—10% of cerebral palsied individuals have ataxic involvement resulting from involvement of the cerebellum. Common to ataxia are weakness, uncoordination, poor balance, wide base gait, and difficulty in rapid and fine movements.
- *Mixed*—This form of cerebral palsy is the most common form. Rarely is any one individual spastic, athetoid, or ataxic alone. Most often you will

see spastic athetoids and less often ataxic athetoids. This category of involvement presents the reasoning for the large variability of motor involvement
seen in CP.

The following terms describe CP affecting various body areas:

- *Quadriplegia*—Muscular involvement of all four extremities and trunk. Up-
  per extremities are usually more involved than lowers.
- *Triplegia*—Muscular involvement in three extremities and trunk.
- *Diplegia*—Two lower extremities much worse than upper extremities.
- *Paraplegia*—Essentially two extremities involved, usually lowers, with min-
  imal upper extremity involvement (mild form of diplegia).
- *Hemiplegia*—Usually involves one upper extremity and one lower extremity
  on the same side (upper extremity usually worse).
- *Monoplegia*—One extremity involved (may be considered mild hemiplegia).

With regard to the medical versus functional classification issue, CP experts
favor the functional approach. Not only is this classification system disability specific, but it is also sports specific, with each athlete assigned a classification for
track, field, and swimming separately. Most athletes end up with the same classification for these three events, but approximately 15% have split classifications
(e.g., Class III in track but Class IV in field). When this occurs, and one classification must be used for all athletes as in research, the track classification is believed
to be the most indicative of overall functional ability. Horseback riding entails
a slightly different classification system with placements more similar to swimming than to track or field. The classification portion of the *Rules Manual* stresses
the following:

> An important point to conceptualize about the classification process is that
> two athletes may have the same *functional ability*, but the quality of their
> *performance* may differ due to better technique and conditioning. Also, it
> is conceivable that an athlete may improve his/her functional ability because
> of vigorous participation in sport and, therefore, necessitate a possible change
> in classification. (NASCP, 1983, p. 14)

A description of the sport classification used by the United States Cerebral Palsy
Athletic Association (USCPAA), as well as Cerebral Palsy–International Sports
and Recreation Association (CP-ISRA), is presented in summary form in Table 1.

Associated Dysfunction

Much of the rationale for the disability specific classification system in CP sports
pertains to the prevalence of associated dysfunctions that occur in conjunction
with upper motor neuron lesions. Unlike spinal cord injured athletes and competitors whose disabilities affect only strength, balance, and range of motion of lower
extremities, persons with CP typically have to cope with abnormal reflex activity
and muscle tone, perceptual-motor problems, visual dysfunction, learning disabilities, and other soft signs of neurological damage such as attentional deficits, hyper-

Table 1   Sports Classification System

Class I	Severe involvement in all four limbs. Limited trunk control, unable to grasp a softball. Poor functional strength in upper extremities, necessitating the use of an electric wheelchair.	**Class V**	Good functional strength and minimal control problems in upper extremities. May walk with or without aides, but for ambulatory support.
Class II	Severe to moderate quadriplegic, normally able to propel wheelchair with legs or if able, propel wheelchair very slowly with arms. Poor functional strength and severe control problems in the upper extremities.	**Class VI**	Moderate to severe quadriplegic. Ambulates without walking aids, less coordination balance problems when running or throwing. Has greater upper extremity involvement.
Class III	Moderate quadriplegic, fair functional strength and moderate control problems in upper extremities and torso. Uses wheelchair.	**Class VII**	Moderate to minimal hemiplegic. Good functional ability in nonaffected side. Walks/runs with a limp.
Class IV	Lower limbs have moderate to severe involvement. Good functional strength and minimal control problems in the upper extremities and torso. Uses wheelchair.	**Class VIII**	Minimally affected hemiplegic. May have minimal coordination problems. Able to run and jump freely. Has good balance.

Note. From *International Games for the Disabled. Official Program for 1984* (p. 20) by F. Koch, 1984, Nassau County, NY: Author. Reprinted by permission.

kinesis, and impulsivity (Bleck & Nagel, 1982; Sherrill, 1981; Thompson, Rubin, & Bilenker, 1983). Although these problems are not discussed in current CP-ISRA and USCPAA manuals, official classifiers are trained to observe and take them into consideration when making classification judgments.

It has been estimated that 88% of the general CP population has three or more disabilities (Thompson et al., 1983). Although much has been published on the general CP population in regard to associated dysfunctions, little is known about CP athletes as a specific subpopulation. The major difference between the general CP population and the CP athlete subpopulation seems to be cognitive functioning. Current texts state that 30 to 70% of the general CP population have mental retardation (Bleck & Nagel, 1982; Levine, Carey, Crocker, & Gross, 1983; Thompson et al., 1983). In marked contrast to this, CP sports experts indicate that only 10 to 15% of USCPAA athletes have mental retardation (Sherrill & Adams-Mushett, 1984). The performance qualifying standards for national and international CP competition are such that few persons with both CP and mental retardation can demonstrate the times and distance required for inclusion in sports events. The 1983 *NASCP Manual* (p. 11) states specifically that CP sports are for athletes who are not eligible for Special Olympics (i.e., persons with CP who demonstrate average or better intellectual functioning). Current assessment theory emphasizes the difficulties in accurately determining the IQs of severely disabled cerebral palsied persons, however, and much work is needed in this area. Many persons with CP, previously considered mentally retarded because of communication and other disorders, are now believed to have IQs within the average range.

Newer texts (Thompson et al., 1983) are beginning to stress learning disabilities rather than mental retardation as characteristic of much of the general CP population. Illustrative of this trend is the following:

Subtle deficiencies in central processing manifest themselves as *an uneven profile* or *scatter* on psychologic testing and as learning dysfunction in the school-age child. In cerebral palsy, scatter is simply a marker of disordered neurologic functioning. In our experience, children who "scatter" seldom do as well as would be predicted by the summary scale. . . . The prevalence of learning dysfunction in cerebral palsy is unknown but appears high. (Thompson et al., 1983, pp. 88–89)

The results shown in Table 2 of a recent study done at Michigan State University during the 1985 National Cerebral Palsy/Les Autres Games support the assumption that many individuals with CP are, indeed, of average intelligence.

In order to contrast the percentage of associated dysfunctions reported for the general CP population with that which seems to characterize the CP athlete sub-

Table 2   Completed Education and Current Employment and Education Status (in % Surveyed)

Highest level of education completed		Current employment and education status	
Elementary school	6	Full-time employment	23
Junior high school	6	Part-time employment	15
Some high school	10	Full-time student	16
High school graduate	29	Part-time student	11
Some vocational school	2	No school or work	32
Some college	26		
College graduate	14		
Graduate school	7		

Note.   This information is based on data collected on 197 athletes, of whom 147 had CP, during the 1985 National CP/LA Games (Dummer, 1986).

population, Sherrill (1984) requested five CP sports experts to estimate percentages of each dysfunction for Classes I to IV and V to VIII athletes. The results of this survey appear in Table 3. To emphasize the difference between CP athletes and the CP general population, these findings are compared with those reported in medical texts.

Concerning visual problems, CP experts estimate that 25% of their athletes are affected. Bleck and Nagel (1982) give no statistics but state that

> many . . . are far sighted (hyperopia); nearsightedness (myopia) is seen mostly in prematures. Crossed eyes (esotropia) are six times more common than turned-out eyes (exotropia). Failure of the upward gaze is characteristic of athetosis due to Rh incompatibility. (p. 71)

Thompson et al. (1983) state that strabismus (crossed eyes) affects approximately 50% of the CP population and is the most common visual disturbance associated with CP. Of CP persons with hemiplegia, 25% have been diagnosed as having homonymous hemianopsia (i.e., blindness in one half of the field of vision, specifically blindness of the nasal half of one eye and the temporal half of the other eye). This condition is usually associated with sensory deficit on the affected side.

With regard to perceptual-motor disorders, CP experts estimate that approximately 60% of their athletes are affected. Problems with spatial relationships (seeing things in a distorted manner) particularly affect staying in lanes during track events, positioning in soccer, and activities requiring targets. Molnar and Taft (1977) stated that 25 to 50% of the pediatric CP population have perceptual deficits. Little research, however, has been conducted on perceptual deficits in CP (Abercrombie, 1964); one reason for this is difficulty in assessing whether the obvious problems are of an input, processing, or output nature.

CP sports experts estimate that about 12% of their athletes have hearing problems. Bleck and Nagel (1982) indicate that only 2% of persons with spasticity

Table 3   Mean Percentages of Associated Dysfunctions in CP Athletes Based on Estimates by Five CP Sports Experts

Associated Dysfunctions	Class I–IV	Class V–VIII	Total
Visual problems	30	20	25
Perceptual disorders	75	50	63
Hearing problems	15	8	12
Learning disabilities	55	40	48
Reflex problems	85	50	68
Seizures	40	20	30
Mental retardation	15	10	13

have hearing problems but that hearing loss is common in persons with athetosis, particularly that caused by rubella or Rh factor incompatibility. Thompson et al. (1983) estimate that 6 to 16% of the CP population is deaf, with kernicteric athetoid children having the greatest incidence (about 60%).

Approximately 30% of CP athletes are believed to have seizures. This is consistent with Thompson et al. (1983), who state that 25 to 35% of children with CP have seizures. In marked contrast, Bleck and Nagel (1982) indicate that convulsive disorders occur in 86% and 12% of persons with spasticity and athetosis, respectively. Molnar and Taft (1977) estimate that 25 to 50% have epilepsy.

Abnormal reflex activity and muscle tone, however, are the greatest problems affecting CP athletes. Almost all (85%) Class I to IV athletes must cope with these, and 50% of Class V to VIII athletes are affected. The reflex problems of CP are well documented (Bobath, 1980; Fiorentino, 1981; Kottke, Stillwell, & Lehmann, 1982), although percentages are seldom stated for adults. Bleck (1975) indicated that 94% of a nonambulatory CP sample retained primitive reflexes into adulthood. Muscle tone abnormalities are hypertonus (i.e., spasticity) and fluctuating hyper- and hypotonus (i.e., athetosis). Asked which type of CP dominated or influenced their sports ability most, 200 national level CP athletes indicated the following: spasticity, 61%; athetosis, 17%; other, 10%; and not applicable, 12% (Sherrill, Rainbolt, & Adams-Mushett, 1984).

Clearly the associated dysfunctions that characterize CP athletes form a strong rationale for disability-specific rather than integrated classifications. Dr. Cairbre McCann, Chair of the Medical Committee of the International Stoke Mandeville Games Federation (ISMGF) and a past member of the advisory committee of the National Association of Sports for Cerebral Palsy (NASCP), summarizes the justification for disability-specific classification as follows:

Speaking as a physician who has witnessed the tremendous difficulties in attempting to match in sports competition cerebral palsied persons and paraplegics or quadriplegics in wheelchairs, it has been evident to me for a long time that in no way can fair competition exist in most cases in which we have attempted to fit the cerebral palsied competitor in the existing classification system (ISMGF). . . . The key element in this testing procedure (ISMGF) is the assessment of strength. Since persons with cerebral palsy may have very adequate strength but poor ability to coordinate or put this strength to use in athletic competition, the result has usually been in the past that the cerebral palsied person found himself (herself) placed in a totally unsuitable and unfair competition so that he (she) usually has been outclassed. (McCann, 1976, p. 19)

Medical and Athletic Training Concerns

When working with any physically disabled population, there is usually a concern over the medical implications of participation in competitive sports. CP is no exception. Experience implies, however, that no additional concerns above the normally imposed first aid/athletic training requirements of a good high school athletic team are required when working with a CP sports team.

Teams are generally recommended to have at least one member of their coaching staff that has athletic training experience and/or at least a Red Cross First Aid Certificate in order to deal with the minor injuries that will occur. Again, injuries, if they occur, will be very similar to those experienced by able-bodied athletes participating in the same sports. Table 4 lists the 32 sport-related injuries that were reported to the medical staff at the 1985 National CP/LA Games, as well as a list of sports that the injuries were attributed to.

One or two physical therapists will also be important when implementing a well-structured warm-up and flexibility program, the first and most important precaution to potential injury.

Some teams include a nurse on their coaching staff to handle the dispensing of medication. Seizure medication is the most common medication used by CP athletes. Medication will play a much more important role with certain les autres athletes due to the variety of associated dysfunctions and often progressive nature of the athlete's disability. Regardless of the disability, it is suggested that medical forms with a section for medications be required from all athletes prior to participation. Side effects and implications of exercise should be cross-referenced with a recent pharmacology text. If there is a question about exercise being contraindicated, contact the athlete's doctor immediately.

Concern for safety and need for minor medical attention in many cases will not be restricted to the practice field. Table 5 lists 32 non-sport-related medical incidences that were also reported during the same 8-day period at the 1985 National CP/LA Games.

A variety of trained staff, a well-outfitted first aid/athletic trainer's kit, appropriate warm-up and cool-down exercises, and a sensible approach to overall safety within your program will be suitable medical precautions for any CP sports program.

Table 4 Incidence of Sport-Related Injuries, 1985 National CP/LA Games

Muscle strains	10	Abrasions	2
Contusions	8	Blisters	1
Bruised elbows	3	Tendinitis	1
Sprained ankles	3	Hand/finger injuries	1
Lacerations	2	Multiple injuries	1

Injuries were attributed to the following sports:

Ambulatory soccer	8	Power lifting	1
Wheelchair soccer	8	Swimming	1
Track events	7	Cycling	1
Field events	3	Equestrian	1
Unknown/unreported	2		

Table 5   Non-Sport-Related Incidences During 1985 National CP/LA Games

Injuries due to falls while walking	16	Bee sting	1
W/C accidents	4	Food in throat	1
Flu symptoms	4	Dizziness	1
Old injuries acquired before Games	2	Chest pain—related to stress	1
Scratch on arm	1	Finger closed in door	1

Other Eligible Disabilities

There are two other disability groups that are eligible to participate in USCPAA competitions. Because loss of motor function is a common residual effect of strokes (cerebrovascular accident—CVA) and closed head injuries that often manifests itself in a similar manner to that of congenitally acquired CP, individuals disabled by strokes or closed head injuries are eligible to participate in USCPAA competition.

Stroke patients, in many cases, will be unlikely candidates for your sports programs simply because of age. However, youth is, unfortunately, not an automatic prevention from having a stroke. Many people today are recovering from the neurological damage of strokes, many of which could gain from the social, emotional, and physical benefits of a well-organized sport program.

A recent emphasis in rehabilitation services has made rehabilitation programs popular for the closed head-injured. Programs range from independent living environments to supported work activities.

Regardless of the type of program, one common problem facing most closed head-injured patients is the need to relearn many previously acquired motor patterns. Similar to an individual who has recently had a stroke, a closed head-injured patient may experience a great deal of frustration because of an inability to do simple tasks that he or she once took for granted. Adapted sports opportunities can provide the stepping stones back to the mainstream of a productive life. Leisure time and the quality use of that leisure time are often a very significant part of an individual's rehabilitation process. When introduced progressively at the proper point in the person's rehabilitation program, sports can provide the positive incentives to encourage progress in all areas of the rehabilitation program. Although sports are not the only part of a person's rehabilitation plan, it certainly can play a significant part when properly integrated into an individual's program plan.

Conclusion

It is almost impossible for us to paint a picture of what a typical CP athlete is going to be like. The information presented here implies there is no such thing as a typical CP athlete, just as there is no typical able-bodied athlete. Anyone who has ever watched or run in either the Boston or New York Marathon can understand this point.

An important thing to remember is that differences set athletes apart from non-athletes, regardless of what segment of the population is being researched: able-bodied, disabled, CP, or spinal cord injured. What should also be understood is that sports and CP are not interchangeable. Not every person with CP will be eagerly awaiting the coach's whistle, just like not every able-bodied person in America has aspirations of being on the next U.S. Olympic Team.

More and more researchers are discovering (as they have with other disability groups) that an athlete is an athlete, regardless of the fact that he or she has CP. More and more of our programs are realizing this and making the transition from a recreationally based program to a competitive sports team, while addressing the individual and varied needs of each athlete on their team. As indicated within this material, a number of associated conditions and individual characteristics may influence an athlete's ability to participate. Certain activities and/or exercises outlined within this manual may, indeed, be contraindicated because of an associated condition. Play it safe; require medical forms, and when in doubt, ask.

References

Abercrombie, M. (1964). *Perceptual and visuomotor disorders in cerebral palsy.* London: Heinemann.

Bleck, E.E. (1975). Locomotor progress in cerebral palsy. *Developmental Medicine and Child Neurology, 17,* 18–24.

Bleck, E.E., & Nagel, D. (Eds.). (1982). *Physically handicapped children: A medical atlas for teachers* (2nd ed.). New York: Grune & Stratton.

Bobath, K. (1980). *A neurophysiological basis for the treatment of cerebral palsy.* London: Heinemann.

Dummer, G., Habeck, R., Ewing, M., & Overton, S. (1986). *A study of athlete participation in the 1985 National Cerebral Palsy/Les Autres Games.* Unpublished manuscript, School of Health Education, Counseling Psychology and Human Performance, Michigan State University, East Lansing.

Fiorentino, M. (1981). *A basis for sensorimotor development—Normal and abnormal.* Springfield, IL: Charles C Thomas.

Koch, F. (1984). Disability classification for competition. In (Ed.), *International Games for the Disabled.* (official program for 1984, p. 20). Nassau County, NY: Author.

Kottke, F., Stillwell, G. K., & Lehmann, J. (1982). *Krusen's handbook of physical medicine and rehabilitation.* Philadelphia: W. B. Saunders.

Levine, M., Carey, W., Crocker, A., & Gross, R. (1983). *Developmental behavioral pediatrics.* Philadelphia: W.B. Saunders.

McCann, C. (1976). Sports activities for the cerebral palsied. *Sports 'N Spokes, 2,* 19–20.

Molnar, G., & Taft, L. (1977). Pediatric rehabilitation. Part I. Cerebral palsy and spinal cord injuries. *Current Problems in Pediatrics, 7,* 28.

National Association of Sports for Cerebral Palsy. (1983). *NASCP-USA classification and rules manual* (2nd ed.). New York: Author.

Sherrill, C. (1981). *Adapted physical education and recreation: A multidisciplinary approach* (2nd ed.). Dubuque, IA: Wm. C. Brown.

Sherrill, C. (1984). *Associated dysfunctions of cerebral palsied athletes*. Unpublished manuscript, Texas Woman's University, Denton.

Sherrill, C., & Adams-Mushett, C. (1984). Fourth national cerebral palsy games: Sports by ability . . . not disability. *Palaestra,* **1,** 24–27, 49–51.

Sherrill, C., Rainbolt, W., & Adams-Mushett, C. (1984). *Characteristics of CP athletes competing in national meets.* Unpublished manuscript, Texas Woman's University, Denton.

Thompson, G., Rubin, I., & Bilenker, R. (Eds.). (1983). *Comprehensive management of cerebral palsy.* New York: Grune & Stratton.

Les Autres Athletes: The Others

Claudine Sherrill
Carol Mushett
Jeffery A. Jones

Les autres, the French term for "the others," is used in sports literature to denote other locomotor disabilities. As mentioned in the opening chapter, les autres athletes have been part of the cerebral palsy (CP) sports movements since its inception. The growth of CP sports has been concurrent with the nationwide emphasis on cross-disability programming. Local sports and recreation programs combine services to provide activities for people with varying disabilities. This, in turn, introduced sports to a segment of the disabled population who had never before had the opportunity to participate. This chapter will take a closer look at the les autres and its relationship to the United States Cerebral Palsy Athletic Association (USCPAA).

Les Autres Disabilities

The brief description of the most common les autres disabilities listed in the *ISOD* (International Sports Organization for the Disabled) *Handbook* (1983) follows.

- *Dwarfs,* better known in the United States as *Little People* because of the efforts of their self-advocacy organization, are medically defined as having short stature (i.e., physical growth that is more than three standard deviations from the mean for the age group). Although many causes of dwarfism have been established (Bleck & Nagel, 1982), the *chondrodystrophies* (defects of endochondral ossification resulting from failure of the skeleton to respond to the normal hormonal growth stimuli) appear most common. Among terms used to specify dwarfism are the skeletal dysplasias, achrondroplasia, and the Morquio syndrome.
- *Osteogenesis imperfecta* (OI) is an inherited condition in which bones are abnormally soft and brittle and therefore break easily. These breaks peak between 2 and 15 years, after which the incidence of fractures is reduced. Characteristics include short stature and small limbs that are bowed in various distortions resulting from repetitive fractures. Joints are hyperextensible with predisposition for dislocation. Most athletes with OI are in wheelchairs.
- *Ehlers-Danlos syndrome* is an inherited condition characterized by hyperextensibility of joints with predisposition for dislocation at shoulder girdle, shoulder, elbow, hip, and knee joints. Other features are loose and/or hyperextensible skin, slow wound healing with inadequate scar tissue, and

19

fragility of blood vessel walls. Smith (1976) states that these persons should be cautioned to avoid traumatic situations.

- *Arthrogryposis multiplex congenita* (AMC) is a nonprogressive congenital contracture syndrome usually characterized by internal rotation at the shoulder joints, elbow extension, pronated forearms, radial flexion of wrists, flexion and outward rotation at the hip joint, and abnormal positions of knees and feet (see Figure 1). Most athletes with AMC are in wheelchairs and have very limited range of motion.

- *Limb deficiencies,* including *dysmelia* (absence of arms or legs) and *phocomelia* (absence of middle segment of a limb, but with intact proximal and distal portions; see Figure 2). In the latter, hands or feet are attached directly to shoulders or hips, respectively. It is sometimes unclear, from casual observation, whether limb deficiencies should be considered as les autres or as congenital amputations. The *ISOD Handbook* (1983) states, for instance, that in swimming, congenital amputations leaving hands or feet intact, in most cases, belong to the amputee classes. The limb deficiency category of les autres was designed for conditions not classifiable within the amputee system.

- *Anisomelia,* referring to a condition of asymmetry between limbs, characterizes many persons who have recovered from poliomyelitis and diseases or injuries that paralyze only one side of the body. The eligibility requirement is at least 7 cm asymmetry for most sports and 10 cm for swimming. In contrast to this ISOD rule, persons with postpolio disability in the U.S. compete with spinal cord injured rather than with les autres athletes.

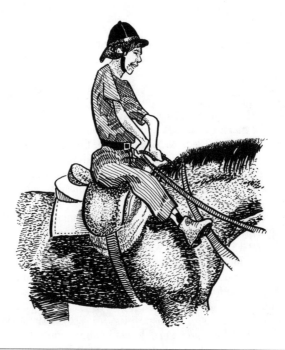

Figure 1.   A young equestrian who has arthrogryposis.

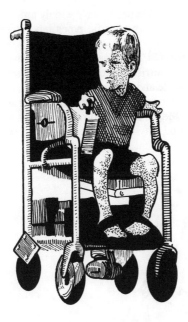

Figure 2.   Les autres athlete with congenital amputations.

- *Ankylosis* is a stiffening or restriction of the normal range of motion of a joint by tissue changes within or without the joint cavity (Brashear & Raney, 1978). It results from chronic arthritis, infection, or trauma, including severe burns about a joint. Among the more common types is *ankylosing spondylitis* (Bechterew disease or chronic arthritis of the sacroiliac joints and lumbar spine).
- *Arthrodesis* (i.e., fusion) is the surgical fixation of a joint used to stabilize a paralyzed or excessively hypotonic limb like a flail (dangle) foot or any joint in which muscle paralysis causes subluxation, dislocation, or complete lack of limb control (Drennan, 1983).
- Conditions characterized by muscle weakness that are caused by peripheral nerve (axon) damage like the Barre-Guillain and Charcot-Marie-Tooth syndromes. *Barre-Guillain* syndrome, a transient condition of muscle weakness, is similar in symptomology to polio (Brashear & Raney, 1978). Recovery is usually complete but may require many months of bracing and therapy; some persons are left with residual muscle and respiratory weakness (Kottke, Stillwell, & Lehmann, 1982). In contrast, there is no recovery from *Charcot-Marie-Tooth* syndrome, which usually occurs between ages 5 to 10 years and progresses very, very slowly (Brashear & Raney, 1978). Clinically, Charcot syndrome begins with involvement of the peroneal (lateral lower leg) muscles and moves slowly upward. Steppage gait (increased flexion of the hip and knee during swing phase) compensates for drop foot caused by peroneal weakness. Eventually upper extremity weakness interferes with throwing and catching activities and fine motor control is diminished. Motor

performance and physical capacity vary widely among persons with Charcot-Marie-Tooth syndrome; six specific types have been identified (Drennan, 1983).

- *Muscular dystrophies* (MD) are genetically determined conditions in which muscular weakness is attributed to changes in muscle fibers (see Figure 3). Muscle cells degenerate and are replaced by fat and fibrous tissue. Most common types are Duchenne, Facio-Scapular-Humeral, and Limb Girdle.
- *Multiple sclerosis* (MS) is a condition described as a demyelinating disease. The myelin sheath (the fatty insulating material that surrounds the nerve fibers

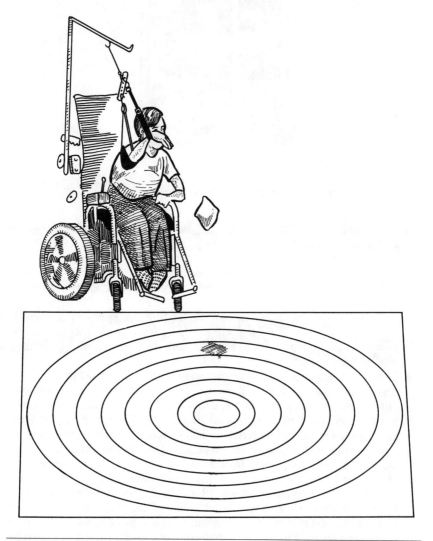

Figure 3. Muscular dystrophy athlete using an arm sling to participate in the precision throw.

of the central nervous system) is somehow destroyed. This results in a short circuiting or blocking of impulses that control bodily function. This demyelinating process is erratic and seemingly very random, leaving the cause and the cure yet unknown. Symptoms can include speech and/or vision difficulties, muscle weakness, numbness, loss of coordination and balance, fatigue, stiffness or spasticity of extremities, and impaired bladder and bowel functions.

• *Friedreich's ataxia* is an inherited condition in which there is progressive degeneration of the sensory nerves of the limbs and trunk (Bleck & Nagel, 1982, pp. 309–312). The most common of the spinocerebellar degenerations, Friedreich's ataxia first occurs between ages 5 to 15 years. The primary characteristics are ataxia (poor balance), clumsiness, and lack of agility, but many associated defects (slurred speech, diminished fine motor control, discoordination and tremor of the upper extremities, vision abnormalities, and skeletal deformities) may develop and affect sports performance. Degeneration may be slow or rapid with many persons becoming wheelchair users by their late teens; others may manifest only one or two clinical signs and remain minimally affected throughout their life cycle.

The 12 disabilities defined above are only a portion of the many conditions possibly eligible for les autres competition. Table 1 lists the 19 different les autres disabilities that participated in the 1985 National Cerebral Palsy/Les Autres Games. The 1985 Games represented the first national sports competition in which les autres were allowed to participate on a nonintegrated basis; les autres against les autres.

Since the 1985 National CP/LA Games, two national organizations have been formed to address the specific needs of les autres athletes. Both, the United States Les Autres Sports Association (USLASA) and the Dwarf Athletic Association of America (DAAA), spun off the enthusiasm established in 1985.

Table 1   Les Autres Disabilities at the 1985 National CP/LA Games

Dwarfism	29	Bilateral AK amp. bilateral phocomedia	1
Muscular dystrophy	16	Charcot-Marie-Tooth disease	1
Arthrogryposis	12	Dystonia musculorum deformans	1
Friedreich's ataxia	5	Fiberous dysplasia	1
Multiple sclerosis	4	Wohlfart Kugelburg-Welander disease	1
Osteogenesis imperfecta	4	McCune Albright syndrome	1
Ehlers Danlos syndrome	2	Myelodysplasia	1
Arterrovenous malformation of the spine	1	Multiple hereditary exosteses	1
Ataxia telagieotasia	1	Tar syndrome	1
		Werdnig Hoffman disease	1
		Total	84

Both organizations are grass-root athlete-organized associations. The Dwarf Athletic Association has a parent association in the Little People of America, Inc. (LPA), a national organization that is comprised of several major regional chapters. The LPA meets annually at the LPA National Convention, which in 1986 provided the ideal opportunity to host the first International Dwarf Games. Competition was held in golf, power lifting, track and field, swimming, table tennis, and basketball. More than 125 athletes participated, including athletes from Canada and Sweden. Plans have already been made to include sports as part of all future LPA conventions.

USLASA, at this point in their development, has chosen to work cooperatively with USCPAA and participate in a combined national event as they did in 1985.

International competition for les autres is governed by the International Sports Organization for the Disabled (ISOD), which also governs international sports for amputee athletes. This adds more confusion to the issue, for the only United States member to ISOD at this time is the United States Amputee Athletic Association (USAAA). This requires the les autres organizations that compete separately or with USCPAA to negotiate their international representation through the U.S. Amputee Association. Although USLASA has already opened formal communications with ISOD, it is unlikely that official membership to ISOD will be granted until the United States counterpart for les autres sports has grown both in size and independence from USCPAA.

Classification

ISOD, like Cerebral Palsy–International Sports and Recreation Association (CP-ISRA), presents a functional profile against which athletes are compared. A difference between ISOD and CP-ISRA is the extent to which the two organizations believe in sport-specific versus sport-general classifications. CP-ISRA assigns athletes three general classifications: *track*, which is used also for slalom, soccer, bowling, bicycling, and tricycling; *field*, which is used also for archery, riflery, table tennis, and weight lifting; and *swimming*, which is generalized to horseback riding. In contrast, ISOD offers functional profile descriptions for each of their 18 sports: air pistol, air rifle, archery, field, lawn bowling, swimming, table tennis, track, volleyball sitting, volleyball standing, weight lifting, alpine and nordic skiing, biathlon (10-km track and air rifle), Nordic sledge, downhill sledge, sledge racing, and sledge hockey. The sports ability classifications used for track and field by ISOD are presented in summary form in Table 2.

Conclusion

The purpose for including this section was to make the reader aware of the wide variety of disabling conditions that might realistically be represented in a local community-based sports program. It also should emphasize that many les autres athletes, like CP athletes, are affected by a number of associated dysfunctions. Tremendous individual differences characterize the les autres disabilities as well as the athletes themselves. Contraindications in respect to sports participation will

Table 2   Track and Field Classifications for Les Autres Athletes

L1. Wheelchair bound. Reduced functions of muscle strength, and/or spasticity in throwing arm. Poor sitting balance.

L2. Wheelchair bound with normal function in throwing arm and poor to moderate sitting balance. Or, reduced function in throwing arm, but good sitting balance.

L3. Wheelchair bound with normal arm function and good sitting balance.

L4. Ambulant with or without crutches and braces; or problems with the balance together with reduced function in throwing arm. Throw can be done from a standstill or moving position.

L5. Ambulant with normal arm function in throwing arm. Reduced function in lower extremities or balance problem. Throws can be done from a standstill or moving position.

L6. Ambulant with normal upper extremity function in throwing arm and minimal trunk or lower extremity disability. A participant in this class must be able to demonstrate a locomotor disability that clearly gives him or her a disadvantage in throwing events compared to able-bodied sports men and women (Koch, 1984).

also vary from disability to disability and athlete to athlete. Implementation of coaching techniques outlined throughout this manual may or may not be appropriate for a given les autres athlete.

As coaches and program administrators, we cannot afford to take things at face value. Physical examinations prior to participation and ongoing consultation with the athlete's family doctor and physical therapist are common practice in most successful programs. The les autres sports movement is a young and enthusiastic approach to sports opportunities for individuals with disabilities who in the past have had little or no opportunity to participate. In many ways it is a reflection of what occurred 10 years ago with CP sports. With the right direction and support, les autres may someday gain the size and independence they so dearly desire.

Note

For more information, contact: International Sports Organization for The Disabled, Sports Technical Officer, c/o Svenska Handikappidrottsforbundet, Irottens Hus, S-12387 Farstra, Sweden, Telephone: 08-713-60-00 or Dwarf Athletic Association of America, c/o Len Sawisch, 3725 West Holmes, Lansing, MI 48911, (517) 393-3116, or United States Les Autres Sports Association, c/o Dave Stephenson, Greater Houston Athletic Association for the Physically Disabled, 5631 Alder, Apt. 7, Houston, TX 77081, (713) 664-9007.

References

Bleck, E. E., & Nagel, D. (Eds.). (1982). *Physically handicapped children: A medical atlas for teachers* (2nd ed.). New York: Grune & Stratton.

Brashear, H. R., & Raney, R. B. (1978). *Shand's handbook of orthopaedic surgery* (9th ed.). St. Louis: C.V. Mosby.

Drennan, J. (1983). *Orthopaedic management of neuromuscular disorders*. Philadelphia: J.B. Lippincott.

International Sports Organization for the Disabled (1983). *ISOD handbook*. Farsta, Sweden: Author.

Koch, F. (1984). Disability classifications for competition. In *International games for the disabled* (official program for 1984, p. 20). Nassau County, NY: Author.

Kottke, F., Stillwell, G.K., & Lehmann, J. (1982). *Krusen's handbook of physical medicine and rehabilitation*. Philadelphia: W.B. Saunders.

Smith, D. (1976). Recognizable patterns of human malformation (2nd ed.). Philadelphia: W.B. Saunders.

Classification for Competition

Grant Peacock

Until the inception of cerebral palsy (CP) sports in the mid-1970s, individuals with CP were medically categorized through the use of two methods: the body part affected (i.e., hemiplegia and diplegia), and the type of muscle involvement (i.e., spastic, athethoid, etc.). This system has its place in the medical world, but presented several problems in respect to competitive sports. Some type of system was needed to equitably group athletes based on functional ability for competition.

Such a system was first introduced at Springfield College in 1976 at one of the first Regional CP Games ever held in the United States. Revised twice since then, our present eight-category classification system is the recognized system used both national and internationally in CP sport competitions.

The following material is meant to serve as an introduction to our present classification system and the process used to determine an athlete's class. This information should give a general understanding of the broad spectrum of functional abilities within our athlete population and the ability to initially differentiate between classes. That understanding should allow a better perspective of United States Cerebral Palsy Athletic Association (USCPAA) programs and the remaining material contained within this manual.

The first basic assumption of the system relates to knowledge. A person who endeavors to classify CP athletes must have a thorough and common base of knowledge involving items such as those addressed in the enclosed article. This base ensures that everyone is dealing with the same basic knowledge.

The procedure itself involves two separate evaluations, a visual evaluation followed (if necessary) by a functional evaluation.

Visual Classification by Functional Profile

The first task of a classifier is to utilize the functional profiles developed for each class and place a competitor into a wheelchair (I to IV) or an ambulatory (V to VIII) category. Then he or she must decide in which two of the four classes an athlete might compete based on their basic observation.

Functional Evaluation

Where the classification is not absolutely clear-cut, a functional evaluation is the next step. It should be done from general gross motor to more specific motor tasks as related to sport, thus giving an objective, rather than subjective, rationale of classification.

Wheelchair or Ambulation

Look at walking, jogging, and sprint pace. During observation, consideration should be given to the effect of the individual's CP on his or her performance. Is balance a factor? Is it affecting synchronization of arms, legs, trunk, and head? Is the control of the wheelchair or the body affected by speed of motion? Often a person's track class can be determined solely by this test.

Lower Extremity, Trunk, Arm, and Hand Tests

For a more specific evaluation, each of the following areas should be looked at:

Lower Extremity.   Range of movement: Is there any limitation, passive or active? If active limits exist in a wheelchair athlete, is his or her classification affected? If limitation exists in an ambulatory athlete, does it affect balance, stride, or compensatory responses to quick, short movements?

Trunk Control.   This is an area often overlooked in wheelchair classes, but it can often be a determining factor. It can also be a factor in Classes V and VI. The two best ways to look at trunk control in wheelchair athletes is first by asking them to actively flex to touch toes and return to upright, or by asking them to simulate a throwing motion and note trunk movement.

Upper Extremity.   Range of movement: Is there any limitation, passive or active? Here, an athlete is asked to simulate arm movement required in competitive wheelchair pushing, running, and throwing. Often the full effects of CP may not be fully seen unless the athlete is performing the movement required in sport.

Hand Control.   Testing basic functional grasps comes first, because static grasp and release must be observable. But, those same grasps must be observed during throwing because they might be affected by arm movements in sport. This is also true in pushing a wheelchair.

The best environment for classifying an athlete is on the practice field or in the gymnasium where time can be taken to consider all aspects relating to functional ability. This process is not as clear-cut and defined as other sports classification systems (i.e., amputee and spinal cord athletes), and it does involve a limited amount of subjective rationale.

Functional Profiles

The following eight functional profiles developed over the past 10 years represent endless hours of classification sessions and countless more time observing athletic performance. It is vitally important that all coaches involved in USCPAA programs develop an understanding for this process by having a basic knowledge of each functional profile.

Class I

The Class I athlete is a severe spastic and/or athetoid with poor functional range of motion and poor strength in all extremities and torso (see Figure 1). He or

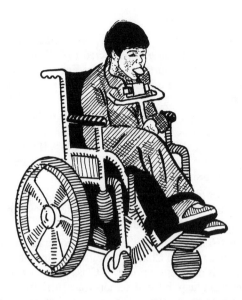

Figure 1.   Class I athlete.

she is dependent on an electric chair or assistance for mobility. The athlete is unable to propel a manual wheelchair because of severe spasticity in the arms and hands.

Lower Extremities.   The Class I athlete is considered nonfunctional in relation to any sport due to severe limitation in range of motion, strength, and/or control. Minimal movement would not change this person's class.

Trunk Control.   Trunk control is very poor to nonexistent when considering frequent shifts in center of gravity requiring volitional compensatory adjustments back to midline or upright position when performing sport movements.

Upper Extremities.   Severe limitation in active range of motion makes this the major factor in all sports. Poor follow-through and shorter throwing motion by up to 50%. Often, only opposition of thumb and one other finger is possible, allowing athlete to grip a beanbag.

Track Classification.   Track classification is determined purely on the lack of independent means of manual self-propulsion other than being pushed or utilizing an electric chair. The only problem arises with someone in an electric chair who has more functional ability in the arms and hands. In this case, hand and arm function should be the determining factor by evaluation.

Field Classification.   Field classification is determined clearly by the lack of hand function to handle club, shot, or discus in conjunction with throwing motion. A person could have somewhat adequate hand function statically, but may have less function when throwing due to athetoid involvement.

Swimming Classification.   Although function may improve or worsen in this area when in the water, evaluation of lack of arm, hand, and leg function should make this class clear.

Class II

The Class II athlete is a severe to moderate spastic and/or athetoid and a severe hemiplegic with fair function in a nonaffected side. They generally have poor functional strength in all extremities and torso. They are able to propel a wheelchair on *flat* surfaces, but have difficulties propelling a wheelchair on an incline slope or uneven surface.

Lower Extremities.   Class II athlete has a demonstrable degree of function of one or two lower extremities, which allows a person to propel his or her wheelchair and automatically qualifies him or her as a Class II lower (Figure 2), unless upper extremity function is more efficient (Figure 3). Often an athlete can ambulate a short distance with assistance.

Trunk Control.   Poor trunk control is apparent during physical exertion in sport, but with training some control can be demonstrated by willpower and resolve, which is often more apparent in water.

Upper Extremities/Hand.   There is severe to moderate limitation. If arm and hand function is as described in Class I, then lower extremity function will determine whether Class II is more appropriate. A Class II upper may not have complete cylindrical or spherical grasp, but can demonstrate sufficient dexterity to manipulate and throw a club, shot, or discus. Throwing motions must be tested for effects on hand function. Wheelchair propulsion with uppers is also demonstrable. Active range of movement is moderate to severe; thus hand function is the key.

Track Classification.   In some cases, if an athlete can propel a chair with arm *and* legs, a choice is made by the athlete. If arm function with hand control when propelling a chair is possible, Class II upper is the lowest class available. Use of an electric chair should not determine the athlete's classification.

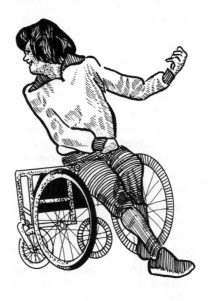

Figure 2.   Class II lower extremity athlete.

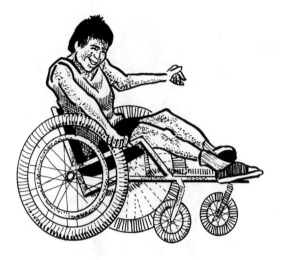

Figure 3.   Class II upper extremity athlete.

Field Classification.   If arms and legs both show sufficient function to enable upper or lower extremity event, they may choose both upper and lower extremity events. If significantly full hand grasp and some trunk movements are observed while throwing, placement in Class III may be indicated.

Swimming Classification.   Improved upper and lower function and range of movement is seen as compared with Class I. Class II athetoids are able to obtain a coordinated stroke in the water. Class II uppers may have a single arm function movement, with the three other limbs severely spastic. The Class II uppers may also have a two-arm symmetrical movement with severe spasticity in the legs and trunk.

Class III

A Class III athlete is a moderate quadriplegic or triplegic and a moderate hemiplegic with almost full functional strength in dominant upper extremity, and nondominant upper extremity is equal or less (see Figure 4). They can propel wheelchairs independently.

Lower Extremities.   Some demonstrable function can be observed during transfer, short distance walking with assistance, or assistive devices. Lower extremity function does not justify wheelchair propulsion by legs rather than arms. Some function can be a factor in the water. Fatigue usually leads to decreased function.

Trunk.   Fair trunk control is shown while pushing a wheelchair, but often extensor tone renders no forward trunk momentum while pushing a wheelchair forcefully. Some trunk movement can be noted also in throwing for postural correction, but throwing motions are mostly from the arm. This is a major factor in nonambulatory capability.

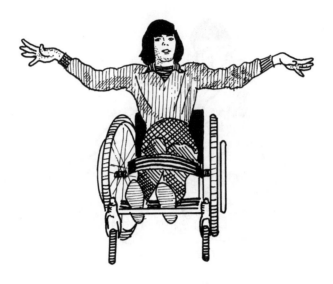

Figure 4.   Class III athlete.

Upper Extremities.   Moderate limitation in dominant arm is usually signified by 25% limitation in extension and follow-through.

Hand Function.   Rapid grasp and release hand movements are usually slow and labored. The dominant hand demonstrates normal grasp of cylindrical and spherical objects, but release on throwing motion or strength of grasp is noticeable less than Class IV.

Track Classification.   Usually some difficulties arise with individuals who show wheelchair mobility and fall functionally between the description of Class III and that of Class IV. The key is trunk mobility in propulsion of a wheelchair, throwing motion, and dexterity in the hands.

If an athlete is unable to use rapid trunk movements with short hand strokes when pushing, he or she is a Class III. In the case of a hemiplegic, one arm may function equal to that of a Class IV, and the only racing class possible is Class III. Less function would raise the question of whether the event is appropriate.

Field Classification.   Often a Class III hemiplegic with near normal function on the dominant side is more appropriate as a Class IV competitor, but a close look should be given to trunk movement. In such a case, this competitor would be a split class performer. In all cases, trunk movement, follow-through, and release are the ultimate considerations.

Swimming Classification.   This is a class that presents some difficulty due to great variability in lower extremity and trunk movement. Generally, as far as upper extremities, this class is clearly more efficient with some rotatory movement bilaterally over Class III, and less so when compared to a IV.

Class IV

The Class IV athlete is a moderate to severe diplegic. He or she has good functional strength and minimal limitation of control problems are noted in the upper extremities and trunk (see Figure 5).

Lower extremities are slow, with moderate to severe limitation, requiring assistive devices for ambulation, with good functional balance.

Lower Extremities. Moderate to severe involvement in both legs, rendering them nonfunctional for ambulation over long distances without the use of assistive devices; a wheelchair is usually the choice of mobility for sport.

Trunk. Accessory trunk movements in both pushing a wheelchair and throwing events are without limitation, with the exception that in some athletes fatigue increases spasticity in the upper portion of posterior part of legs. When standing in sporting events with crutches, this individual usually demonstrates poor balance even with assistive devices, particularly throwing, and has to decide whether to be a Class IV or Class V.

Upper Extremities. The entire upper extremity quarter often shows normal or better strength limits. Some minimal limitation in range of movement may be seen, but a very normal follow-through is observed when pushing a wheelchair or throwing.

Hand Function. Normal cylindrical/spherical opposition and prehensive grasp is seen in all sports. If limitation occurs in upper extremities or hands, it usually is more apparent during a rapid fine motor task.

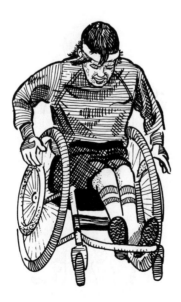

Figure 5. Class IV athlete.

It should be remembered that diplegia implies that spasticity involvement is in all four limbs, with the lower limbs more affected than the upper limbs. Some involvement can always be seen compared to pure *paraplegia* (spinal cord athlete), particularly in functional movement of the hands, arms, and trunk.

Track & Field Classification.   Split classification between Class IV and Class V is often considered a matter of preference for athletes if they are eligible functionally. This is a very competitive class; age, training, and development should be considered. Equipment is also a consideration. Too often a Class IV is dropped to a Class III for inappropriate reasons.

Swimming Classification.   The single greatest problem here is lower extremity and trunk function. Greater function will possibly be seen in the water, making Class IV and V similar.

Class V

The Class V athlete is a moderate to severe diplegic or hemiplegic who chooses to ambulate without a wheelchair in regular daily activities (see Figure 6). This individual may require use of assistive devices in walking beyond short distances, but not necessarily when standing or throwing. An off-center shift of gravity tends to cause the athlete to overbalance.

Lower Extremities.   Moderate to severe involvement of one or both legs may require assistive devices to assist walking. A Class V may have enough function in the legs to participate in Class VI track or insufficient function for Class IV track or Class III track if hemiplegia is present.

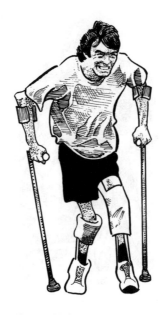

Figure 6. Class V athlete.

Trunk.   When throwing in field events with an assistive device, this individual shows good balance. Without an assistive device, fair to poor balance when throwing is often observed, requiring the athlete to fall within the confines of the throwing area. *This is an important distinction.*

Upper Extremities.   This is an area where variability occurs. Some moderate to minimal limitation in upper extremities can often be seen, particularly when throwing, but strength is within normal limits and often better.

Hand Function.   Normal cylindrical/spherical opposition and prehensive grasp is seen in all sports.

Track & Field Classification.   The major functional difference is trunk balance and function while standing in sport. A Class V *cannot* use a run-up in javelin, whereas a Class VII *can* use a run-up. A wheelchair hemiplegic, Class III, might be a more appropriate placement if single arm function is good but balance is very poor when throwing.

Swimming Classification.   A Class V swimmer has excellent arm and trunk function in water. Lower extremity function, at times, allows the breaststroke leg action and a dolphin kick in the butterfly stroke.

Class VI

The Class VI athlete is a moderate to severe quadriplegic athetoid or ataxic who ambulates without aids (see Figure 7). Athetoid involvement is the most prevalent characteristic in this class.

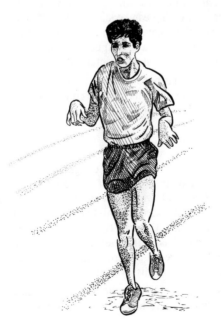

Figure 7.   Class VI athlete.

All four limbs show functional involvement in sport movements. Class VI athletes are very different from Class V. For example, they have mobile spasms that involve alternating movements of lexion and extension, pronation, and supination of arms. Class VI athletes also display asymmetrical tonic neck response activity that produces an asymmetrical postural pattern, which gives a scoliosis with tilting of the pelvis. There is an inward rotation of the hips, producing a lowering of the arches in the feet.

Class VI athletes have more control problems in upper extremities than Class V athletes, whereas Class VI athletes have more function in lower extremities, perhaps not in normal walking, but when running. Internationally, we are witnessing a polarization, and Class VI athletes have now developed into the minimal athetoid group.

This is reasonable because when standing and walking, the above functional profile is adequate, but the athletes themselves perform in a more coordinated way when involved in an athletic skill, for example, running, javelin throwing, or swimming. *Class VI should be for the moderate to minimal athetoid.* These athletes should *not* be placed in Class VII as in previous years.

Lower Extremities and Trunk.   Class VI athletes are functionally better than Class V, but function can vary depending on the sports skill involved, from a poor, labored, slow walking to a running gait that often shows better mechanics. Hence, all Class VI athletes may not be track competitors. There can be a marked contrast between the walking athetoid with uncoordinated gait and the smooth, even-paced, coordinated running action. A run-up in javelin is possible, which is not possible in the diplegic Class V.

Arms and Hand Control.   In the moderate to severe athetoid, control of the hands for grasp and release throwing can be significantly affected when throwing. The more spasticity present, the greater the limits on follow-through and in maintaining balance after throwing. In track, fatigue can increase spasticity in arms and legs, and balance may be difficult to maintain after throwing an implement.

Swimming Classification.   It has become apparent that Class VI swimmers perform in a more coordinated way in water compared to dry land. These competitors can now compete in the breaststroke and may perform a dive start to races.

Class VII

This class is for the true ambulant hemiplegic, congenital or acquired. Class VII has moderate to minimal spasticity in one half of the body. They walk without assistive devices, but spasticity in lower limb causes a marked asymmetrical gait (see Figure 8). They have good functional ability in nonaffected side of body.

The major problem occurs when Class VIII athletes, wrongly classified as being in Class VII, push the true Class VII athletes out. The three types of athletes noted are very comparable in overall athletic function. There has to be a stopping point and some stabilizing of this system.

Lower Extremities.   There is a moderate hemiplegia increase in limb with increased spasticity; noninvolved side has better development and good follow-

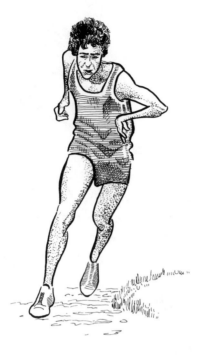

Figure 8.   Class VII athlete.

through movement in walking and running. Running increases spasticity in hemiplegic upper *and* lower limb, causing a marked asymmetrical action. There is a marked difference in stride distance between left and right legs when observed from a lateral position.

When the athlete stands, there is an obvious shortening of the Achilles tendon.

Minimal athetoids should not be placed in this class as previously, but should be in Class VI unless their athetosis is very minimal, in which case they should be in Class VIII. The correct class can only be determined by observing the athlete performing their selected event.

Upper Extremities and Hand Control.   Hand control is usually only a factor in this class in the nondominant hand of the hemiplegic, and some minimal control can be noted with grasp and release, but should not be a factor in competition. The common denominator in upper extremity control is that minimal limitation is seen in the dominant throwing arm.

Swimming Classification.   Class VII athletes can perform a good symmetrical breaststroke arm action and an almost symmetrical leg action. Underwater studies have revealed these symmetrical actions; the only difference from normal is lack of power and propulsion in the hemiplegic side of the body.

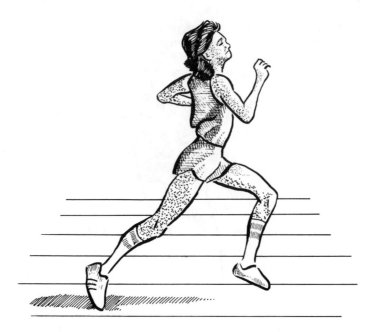

Figure 9.   Class VIII athlete.

Class VIII

This class is for the very minimally involved hemiplegic, the monoplegic (one limb only), the very minimally involved diplegic, and the very minimally involved athetoid (see Figure 9). Consult world records and qualifying standards for guidance.

Class VIII athletes can run and jump freely without a limp. Their gait is symmetrical when walking and running. Class VIII athletes always run with an even stride (symmetrical), compared to the obvious Class VII person who has marked signs of hemiplegia as described in the Class VII functional profile.

These athletes may have minimal loss of full function caused by incoordination, usually seen in the hands; perhaps a slight loss of coordination in one leg, or minimal shortening of the Achilles tendon.

Swimming Classification.   A Class VIII swimmer has good symmetrical control in all swimming strokes and good upper extremity and trunk control in water.

A monoplegic with considerable lack of power in the affected limb may be classified as a Class VII for swimming but a Class VIII for track and field.

Certification of Classifiers

To maintain credibility within the system, classifiers must be certified by USCPAA (as of the 1983 National Games). Criteria for certification is as follows:

1. A degree in physical therapy, occupational therapy, adapted physical education, recreation therapy, special education, or a resumé with specific background applicable to disabled sports
2. Involvement in a USCPAA classification seminar
3. Completion of a written examination relating to medical aspects of CP and specifics of the USCPAA classification system
4. Demonstrated practical ability in administration and interpretation of testing procedures as well as functional profile

Through the implementation of this program, the number of nationally certified classifiers has steadily increased. Programs interested in cohosting a classification seminar should contact the USCPAA representative in their area.

Part II

Training and Preparation

The Role of the Physical Therapist in Exercise Programs

Barbara Cancilla
Marilyn Pink

Those of you who have worked with a physical therapist are aware of his or her knowledge of human anatomy and physiology. As you begin to exercise, your body's anatomical and physiological systems play key roles. Any alterations in these systems may require special considerations, and you can benefit from the analysis and input of the physical therapist. The physical therapist can uniquely contribute to five areas in exercise programs:

1. Educating people with cerebral palsy (CP) in the importance of fitness
2. Evaluating the individual's physical abilities
3. Assisting in developing appropriate goals and programs for the individual based upon the above
4. Instructing the individual in the components of a fitness program, the skills of the activity, injury prevention, and progression
5. Following through with the fitness program

Education

Why should you spend time and energy to be fit? Doesn't the extra energy you spend in dressing and in mobility make you fit enough? Don't you need to be just fit enough to get through all your daily activities? How does fitness benefit you? In order for any activity to be pursued, either you must believe in some future personal benefit, or the activity must be fun. In other words, you must be motivated.

One of the proven ways to motivate people is to educate them in the importance of the activity so that they see a personal benefit. The physical therapist can share scientific data on the general physical, mental, and emotional benefits of exercise with emphasis on the benefits that meet your specific needs. As you learn about these benefits you begin sharing this scientific information with your family and friends. You begin to have a basis for reading and evaluating layman exercise literature, and begin to more appropriately apply this outside information to yourself.

Evaluation

It is necessary to learn about your muscle strength, spasticity, limitations in your joints, and the response of your heart and lungs to exercise in order to develop a safe program. This is done to determine limits and to set a performance baseline. This evaluation is done not only upon initiating the program, but also at predetermined future dates. In addition, a history is taken during the evaluation to identify any prior injuries, as well as to identify your interests.

Developing Goals

Based upon the results of the evaluation, your goals and programs are developed. This history taken during the evaluation will narrow down the area of the fitness activity. The evaluation will specify the activity and realistic expectations. Measurable goals are realistically set with you and the physical therapist. Both short-term and long-term goals are determined. Examples of short-term goals are to swim half the length of the pool on the back with a flotation device in 6 weeks or to be able to consistently serve a racquetball three out of five times from the wheelchair in 4 weeks. Examples of long-term goals may be to complete all stations of an exercise course within 1/2 hour in 6 weeks, or to consistently reach and maintain your exercise heart rate during an aerobic dance class in 4 months.

The programs will include the stretching, warm-up, peak, and cool-down exercises. They can include interval training as well as endurance training. They may include different activities on different days of the week. For example, Monday and Friday may be wheelchair basketball games and Wednesdays may be weight training. The realistic goals and the diversely structured programs can help motivate you to carry out your exercise program.

Instruction

The three major types of exercise (stretching, strengthening, and endurance) are outlined for you. The separate goals of each of these and how the three work together for optimal benefits are explained. The five necessary steps for each workout are discussed (preactivity stretching, warm-up, peak, cool-down, and postactivity stretching). You are told why each of these steps are necessary. By designating the number of minutes per session, the time of day, and the days of the week, you will begin to see the program as realistic and see some structure. This structure helps you to follow through with a commitment to exercise.

Skills of the Activity

In order to be successful in an activity, you must develop new skills. Because of your altered anatomical and physiological systems, the application of the skills may be different. You and your therapist will go through problem-solving techniques in order to design the best skills for you.

Heart Rate Monitoring

Your heart rate is one of the most feasible and accurate indices you can measure that reflects how your heart is responding to exercise. It is simply telling you how fast your heart is beating. As you exercise, your heart has to beat faster in order to get ample blood to your exercising muscles. As you cool down, your heart rate begins to decrease. Your therapist will teach you how to take your heart rate and what your expected heart rate is for each of the aforementioned steps in an exercise program. In addition, your therapist can teach you what symptoms to note, and whom to notify in the event of abnormal levels.

The therapist can also instruct you in a system to document your heart rate and program. In this way, changes can be better followed and interpreted.

Injury Prevention

Your therapist is able to teach you how to prevent injuries while doing your fitness program. Some of the general areas in injury prevention include proper stretching, strengthening weak muscles in order to obtain balanced musculature about a joint, and exercising within your given heart rate parameters. The specific injury prevention depends upon your fitness activity. Here again, your therapist will be able to guide you.

Progression

A participant must know when and how to progress his or her fitness program. Understanding the interrelationship of the various body systems is helpful in understanding the "when" and "how" of progressing. The outcome of the interrelationship is that the body will progress only as fast as the slowest body system. Your therapist can teach you when to progress your program and how to progress it.

Follow-Through

Once you become independent with your fitness program, your therapist can follow through with your progress by occasional phone calls, check-ups or drop-ins. The follow-up is important to ensure the highest quality program has been developed and to troubleshoot for any new problems. A better follow-through service can be provided when you have documented your program and your heart rate response.

Conclusion

As you begin your exercise program, it is important that steps are taken to ensure your safety with the program. Your physical therapist can assist in developing your program by educating you on the importance of exercises, evaluating your physical abilities, developing appropriate goals and programs with you, instructing you in the components of the program, the skills of the activity, injury prevention, and progression, and by following through with your program.

General Sports Training for Individuals With Cerebral Palsy

Alfred Morris

The most important thing when considering overall guidelines or universal rules of training for the athlete with cerebral palsy (CP) is to realize that there are many more similarities among all athletes, even those with certain physical disabilities, than dissimilarities between individuals with handicapping conditions. The point to be emphasized is that principles of endurance conditioning should be applied to any athlete who is training for the Olympic marathon, whether that athlete is able-bodied, blind, deaf, or even cerebral palsied. Principles of endurance training involve long, steady, continuous physical activities of a large muscle nature. Similar rationale could be employed for strength training. In order to participate successfully in a strength activity, one must make muscles stronger. By engaging in proper, variable resistance exercises, the size and strength of muscles can be increased. This will help performance in any physical activity involving strength.

Having said this, what will follow will be cardinal rules of training that will apply to CP athletes wishing to improve their performance.

The Athlete

Before discussing cardinal principles of training, a word must be said about the athlete. The athlete is a gifted individual. The person who is striving to perform his or her utmost in an athletic event is an individual worthy of admiration. They are willing to risk the uncertainties of athletic competition in order to grow as individuals. By daily training and striving toward a goal, the athlete has a reason for being, which many individuals in our society fail to find. With proper, intelligent training and conditioning, athletes can see improvements, learn more about their bodies, and become more physiologically and psychologically healthy as human beings. The athlete learns about sacrifices, effort, winning, and losing, and realizes that perhaps in the end, one of the greatest outcomes of sports and athletics is striving toward a goal. Many times, this journey to achieve a goal is more meaningful than the first place medal itself, in a certain competition.

Now, let us turn our attention to the cardinal rules of physical training and conditioning for sports competition.

Principles of Training

It is important that the athlete always keep uppermost in the mind the overall goal or objective of sports competition. If the goal is to run a long distance endurance race, then training must be directed toward that endurance goal. If the athlete is a thrower of a discus, shot, or javelin, then the athlete must design training programs that will improve performance in that specific event. Training is highly *specific*, as we shall see with Principle 2. The athlete must set daily, weekly, monthly, and even yearly goals in order to be successful in his or her event. By adhering to the following principles of training, the athlete increases his or her chances of being successful in the chosen sport.

Principle 1: Overload/Stress

Exercise stress occurs in a workout session in which the body is overloaded to the extent that the cardiovascular and muscular skeletal systems are stressed to near maximum. This overload/stress concept relates specifically to the *intensity of effort*. A simple way to measure intensity of effort is to have the athletes monitor their pulse rate as they go through the workout session. Young athletes should be able to achieve maximal or near maximal heart rates of 170 to 200 beats per minute. If the athlete is involved in a strength training session, maximal or near maximal weights must be attempted to be lifted with each workout session. These are two examples, one in an endurance workout, and one in a strength workout, of the principle of overload/stress.

Principle 2: Specificity of Training

This specificity of training principle states that athletic training must be highly specific to the sport and to the particular requirements and strategies of that sport. An athlete who wishes to become a tennis player must practice all elements and participate in the sport of tennis. An athlete wishing to become a basketball player must play basketball (all aspects of basketball—offense, defense, foul shooting, etc.). To become a better runner or swimmer, the athlete must run or swim. In addition, there are other strategies that the athlete must follow. If a specific athlete's event is the 800-m run, then in running, this athlete must practice at distances slightly shorter (200 m to 400 m) than the actual event, but also, on certain other training days, must engage in runs of longer distances (1,500 m to 5,000 m) in order to prepare for the 800 m event. One should work several days per week at race pace, the desired pace that the athlete hopes to achieve in the race. If one is working toward a 2:10 800-m time, then the athlete must practice repeat 400 m at 60 to 65 seconds.

Specificity of training involves doing, in practice and training, as many of the activities as are required in as near the same form as the actual competition. This is a simple principle, yet one that is often overlooked in athletic training.

Principle 3: The Training Principle of Progression

This training principle emphasizes that the athlete must work progressively in the overall training program for weeks, months, and perhaps even years, if improvement is to be gained. The first training principle emphasized overload/stress, and related to intensity of effort. Another way of looking at this is the extended *duration* of the effort. In early training sessions the athlete may only be able to work out 15 to 25 consecutive minutes. Using running as an example, the runs in the early part of the seasonal training may only be 15 to 25 minutes at a time. By reducing the effort, the duration of this running activity can be extended by 10 to 25 min, so that the athlete may be approaching a conditioning level where he or she can work approximately 1 h at a time, nonstop.

Principle 4: Recovery and Rest

Athletes cannot work every day at an intense level. We know that certain muscles need rest, and the fuel supply for the muscle (muscle glycogen) must be replenished. This process takes 24 to 48 hours. Severe training days must be followed by rest or very light training days. Signs of overtraining are an elevated resting heart rate in the morning, changes in the appetite, faulty sleep patterns, and general irritability.

Principle 5: Diminishing Returns

This principle indicates that as the athlete continues improvement in training, modest to good improvement will result initially. However, as the athlete continues to train beyond a period of weeks and months and perhaps even for years, he or she will be getting closer to the maximal potential, and therefore, the rate of improvement tends to level off. This is indicated in Figure 1.

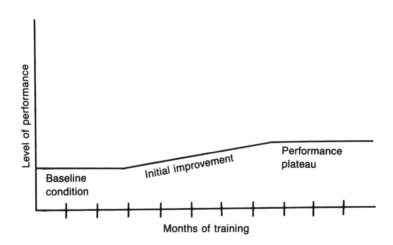

Figure 1. The principle of diminishing returns. From a baseline condition the athlete may make marked improvements during the first several months of training until a plateau is reached. After this point, only intelligent training will cause the athlete to continue to improve at a much slower rate.

Principle 6: Individuality

This final training principle of individuality means that although a group of athletes of the same sex and relatively same age, height, and weight may receive the same athletic conditioning program, the rate of improvement and development may be dissimilar. There are several reasons for this. They may include variations in genetic makeup of each athlete; also, rest, diet, and relaxation schedules may be different. Body build, which is related to genetic type, may be different. The wise coach and athlete realize that there is much variability in characteristics and consequently, must tailor training programs to the individual in order to achieve maximum results.

Summary

The athlete who hopes to improve and increase athletic performance must pay close attention to the training principles outlined above. Although the principles listed above are not all-inclusive, certainly they are the most important ones. The athlete who follows these training principles can expect reasonable improvement and success in sport activity.

Additional Reading

Morris, A.F. (1984). *Sports medicine: Prevention of athletic injuries*. Dubuque, IA: Wm. C. Brown.

Exercise for Fitness

Marilyn Pink

Being fit enables you to be more physically and mentally alert, as well as be more emotionally stable. Studies have proven that individuals who exercise regularly are able to attend to sedentary as well as physical activities for longer periods of time. These people are able to concentrate better. In addition, they tend to be happier. Experiments have been done on depressed people in mental hospitals. Those who were on a regular exercise program decreased their depression without medication. Those not on an exercise program required medication and still were not successful decreasing their depression.

Longevity of life is another bonus for fit people. When the heart, lungs, and muscles work harder, they learn to work more efficiently. The heart becomes stronger and larger. This allows a greater amount of blood and oxygen to reach the muscles with fewer beats of the heart. This is why your resting heart rate/pulse starts to decrease as you become more fit. The amount of oxygen that can be used by the body is increased. Thus energy is conserved and muscle fatigue is delayed. When machinery (including your heart, lungs, and muscles) works more efficiently, it can work longer. This makes sense!

Getting Fit

The first thing you need to know is the skills of the exercise you choose. Once you have chosen the area you want to focus on, you can ask the appropriate people to teach you these appropriate skills.

The second thing you need to know is your target rate. Your target rate is the number of beats per minute that your heart should be beating in order to get maximum benefit from a workout. Health professionals can help you establish your target heart rate. This target heart rate is specifically calculated for you based upon the results of an evaluation.

When initiating a fitness program, it is vital that the five steps are incorporated: (a) stretch, (b) warm-up, (c) peak, (d) cool-down, and (e) stretch again. Stretching brings the muscle into its longest position. During a workout, you do a lot of muscle contracting, which shortens the muscles. The stretching before and after the workout helps to balance out the shortening caused by the contractions. Different activities such as swimming, running, and skiing use different combinations for each activity. Also, because your body is different from people without cerebral palsy (CP), and because the exercise technique is adapted for your specific needs, it is important that the stretching is also adapted especially for you.

The warm-up prepares your muscles, heart, and lungs for an increased workload. During the warm-up, your heart has the chance to gradually beat harder and faster, your lungs gradually begin to send oxygen to your muscles a little faster, and your muscles gradually start to contract and relax a little faster.

During the peak activity, your muscles, heart, and lungs are working at their maximum. Your heart rate is high. You are breathing fast. Your muscles are contracting vigorously. You are performing at your optimum!

The cool-down begins the easing off of the workload for the heart, lungs, and muscles. During peak activity your system has been working at an optimum training level. If you completely stop activity after peak exercise, your heart may have difficulty. It has been receiving and pumping lots of blood, and all of a sudden there is very little blood coming back to pump. Thus, your heart's rhythm may be thrown off by the sudden stop.

Stretching after a workout is the most frequently neglected step of a program. It is just as important to stretch after a workout as before. The rationale for stretching before a workout also applies here. In addition, when exercising, your muscles use certain food products for energy to contract. The food products break down in order to be used. The leftover, broken-down food products make lactic acid. The lactic acid builds up in your muscles, and your muscles start to cramp or ache several hours after exercising. The stretching after exercise helps to move the lactic acid out of your muscles and properly eliminates it from your body. The most advantageous time to stretch is right after the cool-down. If your muscles do ache several hours later, the stretching can be reinforced by additional stretching.

It is *imperative* that you follow all five steps in order to safely become and stay physically fit.

Conclusion

Now, here is the catch and the hard work—you must do *regular* exercise. This means the activity must be a *minimum* of 3 times a week for 20 minutes at your target heart rate. I feel that the importance of this and the amount of fun that can be derived balance out the hard work. My beliefs and desires, however, won't make your body do it. You have to believe and understand these things yourself. Make the commitment. You couldn't be doing it for a better reason: yourself!

Interval Training and Record Keeping: Keys to Improved Performance

George S. Brown

A look in record books will reveal a dramatic improvement in individual athletic performances over the past quarter century. What brought about the sudden spurts in physical achievement? Certainly many possible answers to that question exist, but one answer that seems unassailable is the fact that coaches, trainers, therapists, dietitians, and athletes have adapted a more scientific approach to improving human physical performance.

A scientific approach involves method, observation, measurement, record keeping, and evaluation. One scientific approach that has led to great improvement in physical performance is the interval method of training. An interval program is quite methodic; it can be observed, measured, and recorded readily, and it lends itself to evaluation and goal setting.

What Is Interval Training?

Interval training is actually a very common experience. People suddenly decide, for example, that they want to run a mile or two on a regular basis as a way of losing a few pounds. They quickly discover, however, that they cannot run a mile all at once, but they are able to run a bit, walk a bit, and so on until they cover a mile. By repeating the run-walk attempts over a number of weeks, these people are soon able to run a full mile with no walking intervals.

A formal interval training program is very similar to that common experience. In a formal program, the athlete accomplishes in small segments a task that presently cannot be accomplished as a whole. The object of the training is to enable the athlete to put the segments together as a whole.

Take as an example a wheelchair athlete who wants to wheel 400 m in 2 minutes, but who cannot now do so. But the athlete is able to wheel 100 m in 28 seconds. For this athlete, an interval program might consist of doing 100 m in 30 seconds four times with a recovery interval of 3 minutes between hard efforts. Over a period of weeks, the intervals would be shortened step-by-step to perhaps just 10 seconds. At this point, the athlete might well be able to put the parts together and achieve the goal of wheeling 400 m in 2 minutes.

What happens during the weeks of an interval program is that, through the hard efforts and the ever-shortening intervals, the body adapts to the gradually increasing demands being placed on it. The key to carrying out a successful interval program is careful planning and faithful record keeping.

Planning an Interval Program

A successful interval program begins with assessment and goal setting. The planner must know as thoroughly as possible what an athlete is capable of at the time the interval training is to begin. What is the athlete's general state of health? What disabling factors must be considered in training the athlete? How fast can the runner, swimmer, or cyclist cover sprints, middle distances, and long distances at this point? What's the maximum a lifter can press? How far can the athlete hurl a given implement? How quickly does the athlete tire? What is the athlete's attitude toward the kind of hard work that is needed for improvement?

Study of current records and activity trials are necessary to get answers to those questions. Vague recollections or gut reactions won't do. To be safe, several trials held on a number of occasions are called for. Considering all the data and averaging trial data gives the planner the two basic items needed in setting up a productive interval program.

The first item to consider in an interval program is the goal to be achieved. At this point, accurate data are critical. The data helps assure the setting of reasonable goals. The data helps the athlete understand that reasonableness and accept the goal as a step toward a more challenging goal in the future.

The second item to consider, using the data from the trials, is the kind of interval workout that will be most conducive to achieving the goal. This is a difficult task, but if a thorough assessment of the athlete's ability has been done, the task is simplified. If, for example, trial data indicate that an athlete has good stamina, but is limited in basic speed, workouts will have to be planned to focus on the need for using that speed to the greatest advantage, perhaps by doing few repetitions at high intensity with long intervals between. On the other hand, if stamina is a weakness, then many repetitions over a short distance at an easy speed and with short intervals might be most helpful in achieving a goal set for the athlete.

The RITE Variables in an Interval Program

Interval training involves a number of variables. They are repetitions, interval, time, and effort (RITE). *Repetitions* are the number of times an athlete performs a particular effort, such as swimming 25 m six times or throwing an 8-lb shot 20 times. The *effort* is the task being done. The *interval* is the time taken between efforts, and the *time* is the time used for each effort, such as wheeling a distance in 30 seconds or making a lift so many times in 30 seconds.

As an example of how to work with the variables, consider again the athlete whose major weakness is stamina. Let us assume this athlete is a CP Class III wheelchair racer whose best time for 60 m is 24 seconds (0:24) but whose personal record (PR) for 200 m is 1:55.

It seems reasonable to assume that this athlete who can do 60 m in 0:24 should be able to do 200 m in less than 1:30. Interval training could well be the means of achieving that 1:30 goal.

As an easily obtainable first step, however, we might set 1:40 as the first goal. The pace for such a time is 30 seconds per 60 m. That speed should be easy for this athlete. Now, recognizing that stamina is the major problem area, we might choose 10 repetitions of 60 m at a time of 30 seconds per effort, allowing a rather short interval recovery of only 1 minute.

The next step is to put this data into a table that can be used as a record of progress. Table 1 is a hypothetical record of a few workouts for our hypothetical Class III athlete. Note that the table indicates only two interval workouts per week. A good interval program is physically demanding and should, therefore, allow for at least 2 days of recovery between sessions and note that high intensity interval workouts should be curtailed approximately 2 weeks before a serious competition.

Note in Table 1 that only one variable was changed from week to week. Only the recovery interval was changed; the number of repetitions, time for each effort, and the effort itself were kept constant.

Only one variable should be manipulated in an interval program. The variable chosen should be closely related to what the program is aimed at doing. In the example shown in Table 1, the athlete needed stamina, so shortening the interval between easy, achievable efforts seemed a reasonable choice.

Table 1 A Hypothetical Record of Progress

Week/day	Reps	Interval (seconds)	Time (seconds)	Effort (meters)	Performance/comments
1/1	10	60	30	60	27, 28, 31, 30, 29, 31, 30, 32, 27, 30. Done easily. Uneven times indicate need to concentrate on pace.
1/2	10	60	30	60	29, 29, 30, 31, 31, 30, 30, 30, 30, 28. Pace was better. Done easily. May be able to shorten interval.
2/1	10	60	30	60	29, 29, 30, 31, 30, 30, 31, 29, 29, 28. Pace was still good. Done easily. Will shorten interval.
2/2	10	30	30	60	29, 29, 30, 34, 36, 38, 40, 40. Stopped workout. Interval apparently too short. Will try 45 seconds.
3/1	10	45	30	60	

Table 1 also indicates that too drastic a change in a variable may result in a breakdown in performance. Because in this case the interval was short to begin with, it probably would have been wise to have reduced the interval no more than 10 seconds at a time, and perhaps only after a minimum of four successful workouts at each level.

In carrying out an interval program, avoid the urge to rush toward a goal. Remember, if the program is properly conceived, it will be physically demanding. Allow plenty of time for the athlete to adapt to the ever-increasing demands of the program.

How Is the Length of the Interval Determined?

As has been seen, one can work with several variables in laying out an interval program. The variable most frequently manipulated is the recovery interval itself. How long an interval should be allowed? How does one scientifically determine the interval?

A good way to determine the interval for such sports as track or swimming is to use the athlete's heart-rate recovery time. To do this, the first step is to

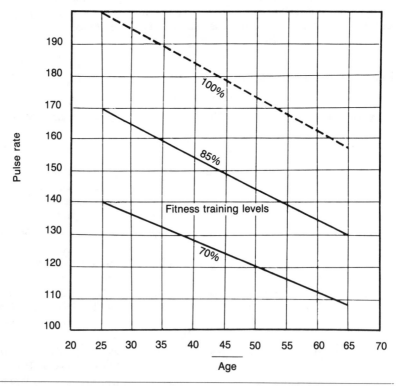

Figure 1.   During hard efforts of an interval workout, a well-conditioned, 30-year-old athlete might have a pulse rate of somewhere between 150 and 190 beats per minute. The interval between hard efforts for this athlete would be as long as it takes for the pulse rate to drop to 75 to 95 beats per minute.

determine the athlete's maximum exercise heart rate. This can be done by having the athlete go all out over a competition distance. Take a 6 second pulse count as soon as the athlete completes the effort. Multiply the number counted by 10 to get the 1 minute pulse rate. You might compare that maximum pulse rate with the age-rate figures shown in Figure 1.

During the hard efforts of an interval program, an athlete's heart rate should reach levels somewhere between three fourths of the exercise maximum and the maximum level itself. The recovery interval between hard efforts should be long enough for the heart rate to drop to about one half of the maximum. For example, an athlete whose maximum exercise heart rate is 200 could easily handle efforts that would generate a heart rate of 150 (three fourths of maximum) to 175. There is a good chance that such an athlete's heart rate would drop to 100 (one half of maximum) in at least 3 minutes—probably less. Thus, for such an athlete, the beginning interval might be set at 3 minutes.

As an athlete gets stronger, the time for the heart rate to drop back to half maximum will decrease. The recovery interval should be decreased to match the improving heart-rate recovery time. Thus, as the cardiovascular system gets more and more efficient, the recovery interval is shortened bit by bit toward the zero point where, theoretically, no interval is needed to accomplish the task.

What Other Variables Can Be Manipulated Effectively?

Although the recovery interval time is the variable most often manipulated in an interval program, it need not be the only one considered. One should remember, however, to change only one of the variables in a particular interval program. The variable chosen should relate to an athlete's particular need. Use weight lifting as an example.

In weight lifting, the mass that muscles can move is the critical factor. It would seem, therefore, that the effort would be the logical variable to manipulate in an interval program designed to help a lifter lift more weight.

In planning an interval program for a weight lifter, one must obviously begin with a weight the lifter can handle easily. Again, three fourths of the maximum seems like a good place to begin. An effort would consist of perhaps five lifts of this "easy" weight. As the athlete improves, the weight is increased until the athlete's current maximum can be lifted those five times. At this point, the athlete should be ready for a new PR.

Table 2 outlines the beginning of an interval program designed to help an athlete who is able to press 100 lb and who wants to reach a new PR of 125 lb. Note that a single effort consists of five lifts of a 75-lb weight in 50 seconds. The athlete then takes a 10 minute interval before beginning the next repetition of lifting the weight five times.

Use of Intervals in Other Sports

Interval training has been used extensively and successfully in running, swimming, and biking. It could clearly be used successfully in weight lifting, but what about other sports such as field events, bowling, and target shooting?

Table 2   A Sample Interval Training Program

Week/day	Reps	Interval (minutes)	Time (seconds)	Effort	Performance/ comments
1/1	3	10	50	5 × 75 lb	Able to do easily. Interval of 10 minutes seems ample. No trouble with three repetitions.
1/2	3	10	50	5 × 75 lb	Handled easily. Will continue as is.
2/1	3	10	50	5 × 75 lb	All goes well.
2/2	3	10	50	5 × 75 lb	OK. Will add 5 pounds to next workout.
3/1	3	10	50	5 × 80 lb	Met challenge well. Did all easily.

At first glance, interval training may not seem specifically applicable to the sports named. A good walking, running, or swimming interval program could do much, however, to improve the overall fitness of any athlete and thus play a contributing role in improving the ability to throw, jump, hit, or shoot. Similarly, a weight lifting interval program could be a useful conditioning tool in many sports other than weight lifting itself.

But, could the interval principle be used to improve throwing, shooting, hitting, and jumping? A creative coach or athlete might be able to apply interval training to some of the sports named. For example, could the use of a vary-weighted table tennis paddle speed up one's arm motion? Could an athlete who throws the shot increase throwing distance by throwing heavier and heavier weights or by throwing more and more times from workout to workout? Could a jumper improve leaping ability by jumping over a low barrier while adding heavier and heavier ankle weights to the legs? Obviously, one would have to be careful to apply such practices to specific muscle groups in ways that would not affect sports techniques adversely.

Record Keeping

Certainly record keeping should be part of any interval work utilized. But there is need for many other kinds of records in a successful sports program. Don't simply limit records to distances thrown or jumped, to scores, to times, to weights, and so on.

One good use of records is to search through them for patterns. Careful records may help you to discover that an athlete's tenth throw or fourth jump is often the best. Put that knowledge to work in practice throws or jumps leading up to competitive throws or jumps. Records may show that one table tennis player may need three or four games to be at his or her best, while another may go downhill right from the start of a game and will, therefore, want to avoid warm-up. Shot-by-shot records may uncover useful patterns for the target shooter. Records may show which splits a bowler needs to work on most.

Careful records that disclose strengths, weaknesses, and patterns can be used to prepare athlete checklists. The athlete runs through the checklist to prepare for competition; the coach uses the checklist to see where the athlete is growing, plateauing, or slipping.

Clearly then, interval training and record keeping as scientific approaches to a sports program can be useful tools. The references cited below, as well as other articles in this book, will be helpful in suggesting other useful ideas in your sports program for the disabled.

Additional Readings

Armbruster, D.A., & Musker, F.F. (1975). *Basic skills in sports for men and women*. St. Louis, MO: C.V. Mosby.

Doherty, J.K. (1980). *Track and field omnibook*. Los Altos, CA: Tafnews Press.

Fox, E.L., & Mathews, D.K. (1974). *Interval training*. Philadelphia, PA: W.B. Saunders.

Katz, J., & Bruning, N.P. (1981). *Swimming for total fitness: A progressive aerobic program*. Garden City, NY: Doubleday.

Murray, J., & Karpovich, P. (1982). *Weight training in athletics*. Englewood Cliffs, NJ: Prentice-Hall.

Flexibility

Karen Rusling

Flexibility should be an essential and valuable component of any athlete's precompetition, competition, and postcompetition season. Regularly done, proper stretching will both sustain and increase an athlete's level of flexibility, prevent injury, decrease the chance of muscle cramping and muscle soreness, and help the athlete to attain individual optimal performance.

Coaches should encourage their athletes to continue regularly on individualized fitness maintenance programs during the off-season. However, for various physiological reasons, many of the athletes will still experience some increase in muscle tightness going into the preseason. It is, therefore, important that the preseason conditioning program emphasize the development of flexibility as well as that of strength and endurance. The stretching exercises during this time are performed at shorter and lower intensities, gradually progressing to longer and more strenuous sessions. Stretching will not only decrease the muscle tightness, but it will also lessen the chances of injury due to overstress as the athlete progresses toward more strenuous training and exercise.

The Three Training Segments

As the training program continues into the season, warm-up, cool-down, and post-workout stretching should become routine for the athletes.

Warm-Up

Physiologically, the warm-up increases the blood supply to the tissues, raising both the general body and deep muscle temperatures. The elasticity (flexibility) of muscles is dependent upon their blood saturation. Cold muscles have low blood saturation, which makes them more prone to injury. The rise in temperature also increases the muscle's ability to accommodate to stress, preventing muscle cramping, muscle soreness, postexercise soreness, or injury to ligaments, muscles, or tendons due to overuse or overstress.

Proper warm-up will stretch the ligaments and other collagenous tissues surrounding the joint(s) in order to increase flexibility.

To begin the warm-up phase, it's best to start with a submaximal activity (such as wheeling or running a couple of slow and easy laps) of about 3 to 5 minutes in duration. Then progress to stretching the muscles, concentrating primarily on the muscles and movements specific to the event or activity.

Without a proper warm-up of at least 15 to 20 minutes, athletes cannot expect their best performance in an event, regardless of how much or how hard they

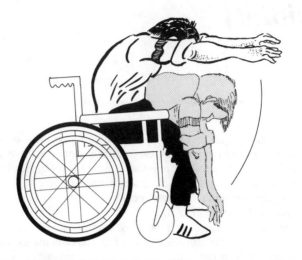

Figure 1.   Toe touch from wheelchair position.

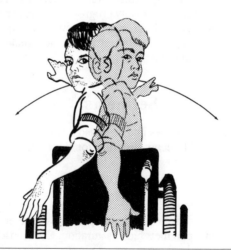

Figure 2.   Trunk twist.

have trained. With a proper and gradual warm-up the muscles, joints, and cardio-vascular system will be primed for maximal flexibility, speed, coordination, power, and endurance.

For optimal benefit from the warm-up, no more than 15 minutes should pass between the completion of warm-up exercises and the actual activity or event. If there are any long periods of time between events (such as in field events) the athlete should do light warm-up exercises during the intervals. On cool days, the warm-up can be increased somewhat in duration. Appropriate sweats or other loose clothing should be worn in order that the body and muscle temperatures are maintained.

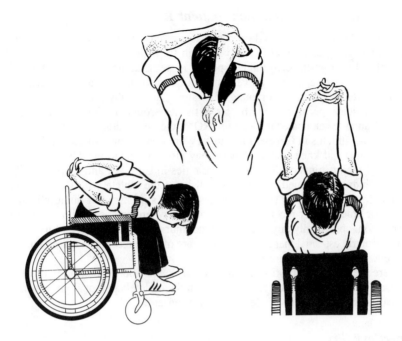

Figure 3.   Upper extremity stretching (3 parts).

Cool-Down

Following any strenuous workout or competition, it is important that the body readjust itself. With a cool-down, the athlete exercises less intensely for a short period of time (5 to 10 minutes) in order to prevent muscle cramping and so that circulation and other body functions will return to their preexertion levels.

Postworkout

For the final phase of the workout, the athlete should repeat the same warm-up stretching routine for at least 10 to 15 minutes. At this point, the muscles are more saturated with blood and are warm, so that additional flexibility is achieved if needed and the incidence of muscle soreness is lessened.

Considerations for Stretching Programs

Flexibility programs should be designed for each athlete's individual needs based on his or her individual limitations in range of motion (ROM) and on the specific events he or she participates in. It is very important that the coach be aware of any and all of the athlete's physical limitations prior to starting him or her on a flexibility or other exercise program.

Common Causes of Limitation to Joint ROM

Muscle weakness will result in decrease or loss of movement. If the muscle is not able to contract (shorten) sufficiently enough to move the part through partial or complete ROM when performing a specific movement, then the ease with which an activity consisting of that movement can be performed is also decreased.

Contractures (permanent shortening of a muscle) are usually caused by increased muscle spasticity, paralysis, or fibrosis of tissues around a joint. The muscle(s) involved cannot be elongated through full ROM, thereby limiting movement. Common in many athletes in Classes I through IV are contractures of the hip flexors, hip adductors, and knee flexors. There may also be limitations due to contractures in all major joints of the upper extremities in Classes I and II specifically.

Many kinds of orthopedic surgeries will leave the athlete with ROM limitations due to adhesions, scar tissue, joint fusions, or stiffness after immobilization in a cast or brace. Other recent medical problems where pain is the limiting factor are common, specifically any athletic-related injuries (muscle pulls, strains, etc.). It is particularly essential that the coach be aware of these recently acquired injuries or recent surgeries so as not to cause further injury.

If there are ever any questions, concerns, or doubts about a flexibility or other exercise program for an athlete, consult with the athlete's personal physician or physical therapist prior to implementing a program.

Hyperflexibility

There is a percentage of athletes (specifically some ataxic CP athletes) who are hypermobile or overflexible. This is a physical characteristic of the individual and not a result of stretching exercises. In contrast to those individuals who may have limitations in their joint ROM, these athletes hyperextend past the "normal" joint ROM. There is a lack of supporting strength around the joints, which can result in decreased strength and increased possibility of dislocation or other damage to the joint structure. An athlete that exhibits hyperflexibility should *not* be put on a flexibility program. In order to perform more efficiently, support of the joints involved is necessary; therefore, they should be put on a program to increase strength and add more stability.

Techniques for Developing Flexibility

Preceding any flexibility program it is essential that the athlete be relaxed. Relaxation through conscious relaxation methods or through deep diaphragmatic breathing are most commonly used. Conscious relaxation of spastic muscles can be achieved to some degree by most athletes. Prior to and following exercise or competition, relaxation can help ensure that there will be stretching of only the connective tissue rather than the muscle fibers, thus eliminating a chance of injury. If the person is very tight and has difficulty relaxing, he or she may benefit from short rest periods before, during, and after the exercise period.

All stretching should be done slowly and with control throughout the ROM. The stretch should be held 10 to 15 seconds without any ballistic (bouncing) movements. Any quick, jerky, bouncing movements will activate the stretch reflex in the muscle being stretched (elongated), causing that muscle to contract (shorten) rather than relax it. Ballistic stretches use the momentum of the body to force the muscles into as much extension as can be tolerated. However, these short-term, vigorous, bouncing movements can cause damage to the muscle fibers and joint structure if this body momentum isn't controlled and/or if there are physiological problems leading to problems in judging how much stretch can be tolerated. So remember, *never bounce;* use slow, controlled stretches and hold.

If the athlete has a muscle spasm during the stretch, hold at that position until the spasm subsides, then continue to stretch past that point.

Passive Stretching Technique

With this stretching technique the athlete does not actively move the body part through the ROM; it is done for them by an outside force. All muscles involved in the passive stretch should be as relaxed as possible (see Figure 4). The motion should be done slowly and very carefully. Caution must be taken with this method because the athlete is not the one controlling the movement or the amount of force used, and injury to joint structures, muscles, or ligaments can occur.

Active-Assistive Technique

Athletes who are not able to complete the full motion actively are encouraged to try and then are assisted throughout the ROM (see Figure 5). With even minimal muscle contraction elicited by the individual some degree of muscle relaxation in the shortened muscle will occur (reciprocal innervation). Once again, caution should be taken to do the motion slowly and with control to avoid injury.

Active Stretching Technique

Many of the athletes in Classes III through VIII should be able to do most of their stretching exercises actively (independently of any outside force). Because no assistance or external resistance is required, these exercises can be performed

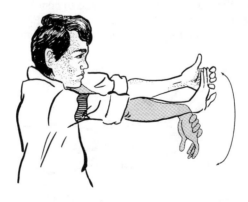

Figure 4.   Wrist stretch through passive technique.

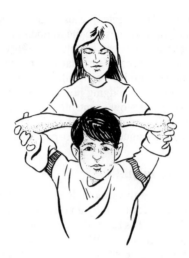

Figure 5.   Shoulder stretch through active-assistive technique.

by the individual at home as well as during training sessions in order to better maintain their current ROM. In contrast to the passive and active-assistive techniques, the athlete is in complete control of the movement. Therefore, with proper instruction and initial supervision, too much force is not likely to be applied, so that injury is prevented.

Proprioceptive Neuromuscular Facilitation (PNF) Relaxation Techniques

PNF relaxation techniques have been proven to be the most successful and recommended methods to use where the goals are to maintain or increase joint ROM. By definition, PNF is a method of improving the neuromuscular mechanism through stimulation of the proprioceptors. ROM is increased by achieving relaxation of the antagonist muscle(s) during the facilitation of the agonist (reciprocal innervation). When the agonist is stimulated to contract, the antagonist relaxes.

Before explaining the specific techniques of the PNF method, a review of a few terms is necessary for a more clear understanding (see also Figure 6).

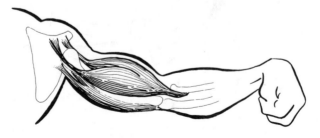

Figure 6.   Agonist versus antagonist muscle.

Agonist.   Prime mover; the muscle that is contracting (shortening); for example, in bending (flexing the elbow), the biceps brachii is the agonist.

Antagonist.   The muscle or group of muscles that oppose the prime mover's action; for example, in bending the elbow, the triceps are the antagonist.

Isotonic Contraction.   Shortening or lengthening of a muscle through its complete ROM (motion occurs; see Figure 7a).

Isometric Contraction.   Contracting the muscles while in a static position; there is no change in the muscle's length; therefore, there is no motion occurring even though the muscle is contracting (see Figure 7b).

Reciprocal Innervation.   Physiologically allows for the smoothness of a movement to occur through the relaxation of the antagonist during the contraction of the agonist.

The following specific techniques are used as substitutes for passive stretching. PNF relaxation techniques are less hazardous and less painful in comparison to passive stretching.

Contract-Relax.   This technique is indicated where spasticity is predominant in the individual and when the person is able to actively move through only part of the range (cannot actively move through the entire range).

The contract-relax method involves the following steps:

1. The trainer, coach, or therapist moves the body part passively to the point of tightness or where resistance is felt (Point A in Figure 8).

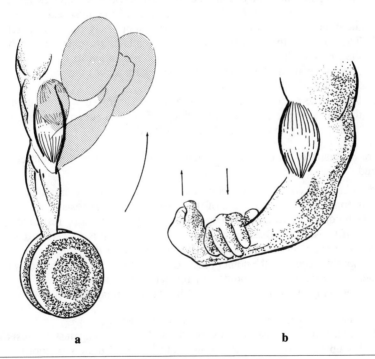

a   b

Figure 7.   Isotonic contraction (a) and isometric contraction (b).

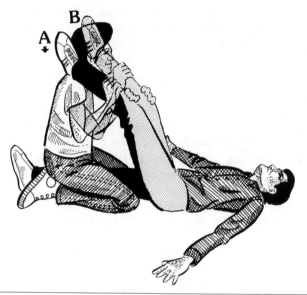

Figure 8.   Contract-relax PNF. Point A is first point on resistance, Point B is ROM gained after relaxation.

2. At this point the athlete is instructed to isotonically contract the antagonist muscle for up to 10 seconds while the coach or therapist resists the movement as strongly as possible (while still supporting the body part).
3. The coach or therapist then instructs the athlete to relax while reducing the pressure (resistance) and waiting for relaxation to occur.
4. After relaxation, the coach or therapist again moves the part passively to the point of limitation (Point B).
5. Repeat the entire procedure several times, followed with an attempt by the athlete to perform the full motion actively without any resistance other than that of gravity or the body part itself.

Figure 8 illustrates an example of a hamstring stretch using the contract-relax method.

Hold-Relax.   In contrast to the contract-relax method, which employed the use of an isotonic muscle contraction of the antagonist against resistance, the hold-relax technique utilizes an isometric contraction at the point of resistance (hold at point of resistance). Because an isometric contraction is involved, there will not be any movement of the body part. It is also the relaxation method used when muscle spasms occur. At the point of the spasm (sometimes accompanied by pain), a coach or therapist should hold until relaxation is achieved.

The following steps are incorporated in the hold-relax method:

1. Passively bring the body part through the ROM.
2. At the point of resistance, instruct the athlete to hold against this resistance for up to 10 seconds (do not let them ''break'' the contraction).

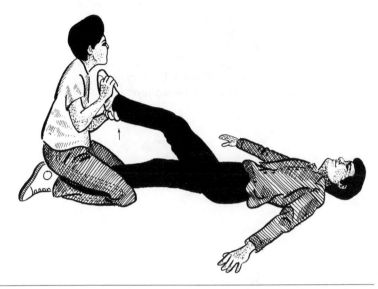

Figure 9.   Hold-relax PNF. Athlete holds against resistance of coach or therapist.

3. Relax, again supporting the body part.
4. Repeat the procedure several times while gently increasing the resistance. Once again, following the procedure, have the person repeat the movement actively without any added resistance.

Figure 9 illustrates the hold-relax method.

Conclusion

A proper flexibility program will certainly improve an athlete's ability to perform a given task. The activities presented within this article represent only a few of the many successful flexibility and stretching techniques and/or exercises. Coaches need to realize that athletes will be the best judge as to the type of exercises that they can or cannot do. Although most athletes should be able to participate in at least a limited stretching routine, it is advisable that coaches consult an athlete's physical therapist and/or doctor before introducing them to a flexibility program. When in doubt, ask.

Additional Readings

Curtis, K. RPT. (1981, September/October). Wheelchair sports medicine. Part 3. Stretching routines. *Sports 'N Spokes,* **7**(3), 16–18.
Daniels, L., & Worthingham, C. (1977). *Therapeutic exercise for body alignment and function* (2nd ed.). Philadelphia: W.B. Saunders.

Klafs, C.E., & Arnheim, D.D. (1977). *Modern principles of athletic training* (4th ed.). St. Louis: C.V. Mosby.

Knot, M., & Voss, D.E. (1968). *P.N.F.—Patterns and techniques* (2nd ed.). New York: Harper and Row.

Pearson, P.H., & Williams, C.E. (1972). *P.T. services in the developmental disabilities*. Springfield, IL: Charles C Thomas.

Strauss, R. M. (Ed.). (1979). *Sports medicine and physiology*. Philadelphia: W.B. Saunders.

Nutrition for Optimal Performance

Alfred Morris

Like many other energy systems, the human body runs on fuel. In order for the athlete to perform, food energy must be converted in the body into muscular energy. Athletes, unlike plants, cannot convert sunlight and soil minerals directly into fuel. The human must get his or her fuel from plant or animal sources. General concepts related to nutrition and how nutrition can affect human physiological performance are discussed here. No matter what specific disability the athlete has, whether he or she be confined to a wheelchair, have some major manifestation of cerebral palsy (CP), or be visually or hearing impaired, the nutrition principles noted below pertain to all people. General principles of nutrition will be listed, together with some suggested guidelines regarding dietary intake, to help the athlete achieve an optimal food intake in order to enhance athletic participation.

Classes of Nutrients

Nutrients are chemical substances found in foods. They function to furnish the body with fuel (calories) in addition to building and repairing body tissue and protecting and regulating certain body processes. There are six classes of nutrients. These classes are listed in Figure 1.

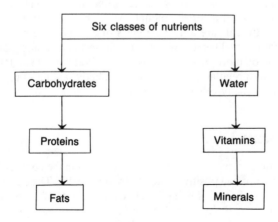

Figure 1. Six classes of nutrients. Carbohydrates, proteins, and fats contain calories, whereas the other three classes do not.

Carbohydrates

Carbohydrates are sugars and starches found in cereals, vegetables, and fruits. In addition, other sugars are added to foods for sweetening (refined sugar, corn starch, etc.). Carbohydrates are the major source for the body, and they are used extensively during severe exercise. Most unprocessed carbohydrates (vegetables, fruits, and whole grains) are rich in food fiber. Fiber is the structural and fibrous element of plants that are essential to a healthy digestive system.

Fats

This nutrient adds flavor and variety to foods and also enhances food taste. Fats provide high energy calories, that is, twice as much energy as proteins and carbohydrates. Fats are found mostly in oils, fatty meats, butter, and other dairy products.

Proteins

After water and perhaps fats, protein is the most plentiful substance in the body. Proteins are broken down in digestion to form amino acids, which are used by the body to repair and build body tissue. Major sources of protein are meats, poultry, fish, milk products, and eggs. Whole grain cereal products, beans, and nuts can also be used as good sources of protein.

These nutrients—carbohydrates, fats, and proteins—provide calories for the body. Carbohydrates provide 4 calories per gram. Proteins also provide 4 cal per gram. Fats, however, contribute 9 cal per gram. A calorie (a large calorie, or kilocalorie) is the amount of heat necessary to raise 1 kg of water 1 °C. Calories are units of energy.

Vitamins, Minerals, and Water

The final three nutrient classes are vitamins, minerals, and water. Vitamins are chemical substances used in small amounts by the body. They serve to regulate body processes. Minerals are a nutrient class of chemical elements essential in small amounts for optimal health. Water is the largest body component. Approximately two thirds or more of the body is water. Water is absolutely necessary because it serves as a regulating substance in the body, aiding in regulating body temperature and in many other body functions.

The American Diet

Diet consists of all food substances regularly consumed in the course of normal living. Optimal diet aims at a positive state of physical health. The current American diet (1980) consists of the following breakdown of foodstuffs: (a) fat, 42%; (b) protein, 12%; and (c) carbohydrate, 46%. What one can observe is that this typical American diet is high in percentage of fat calories. This leads to many degenerative diseases and subnormal human functioning. It is known that large amounts of fat in the diet contribute to cardiovascular disease, cancer of the breast and prostate, atherosclerosis, stroke, diabetes, hypertension, obesity, cancer of the colon and rectum, and possibly appendicitis.

Modifying the diet in such a way that the amount of fat is reduced while carbohydrates are increased is what we call the *Recommended American Diet*. Following the dietary suggestions noted previously, one can lower the percent of fat in the diet while at the same time raising complex carbohydrates. Such a modification might look as follows:

- Fat—32 to 37% (reduction of 5 to 10%)
- Protein—12 to 15% (little or no change)
- Carbohydrate—56% (an increase of 5 to 10%)

The above modification of the diet will reduce fat while increasing carbohydrate intake. Because carbohydrates are used extensively in very intense exercise, this change should enable the athlete to perform better.

A final modification can be made to the diet whereby carbohydrate intake is increased to an even larger degree. Consequently, fats are reduced even more. The suggested American athlete's diet for optimal performance follows:

- Fat—20 to 30%
- Protein—12 to 15%
- Carbohydrate—68 to 55%

Weight Control and Diet

The healthy body uses energy for various metabolic processes. Food (calories) must constantly be supplied for growth and maintenance of body tissue, as well as to maintain body temperature. The largest expenditure of energy occurs as the basal metabolic rate (BMR). The BMR is that necessary resting basal metabolism that is required for cardiovascular function, respiration, and other ongoing body functions. The BMR is highly dependent on sex, age, and body size. As energy expenditure increases during daily activities such as working, going to school, and participating in sport activities, caloric intake must increase.

The fundamental law of nature indicates that there must be a balance of energy intake (food) and energy output (energy expenditure, BMR + other work) in order for weight to be maintained. Creating an imbalance of intake or increase in expenditure distorts this very careful balance and leads to a weight gain or a weight loss (see Figure 2).

The best way to burn excess weight (i.e., excess fat), would be to slightly decrease food intake while increasing energy expenditure in the form of exercise. A person who increases his or her energy expenditure by walking or running 1 mile burns about 100 cal for this exercise. So if one were to run 10 miles over a 3-day period, one could expect to lose approximately 1,000 calories. One has to lose approximately 3,500 cal in order to burn 1 lb of body fat. A general weight loss guideline is that the athlete should lose about 1 lb of body weight (hopefully, all body fat) per week. Drastic weight reduction programs that involve the athlete losing 2 to 4 lb per week can be detrimental. In many of these cases, lean muscle tissue will be lost.

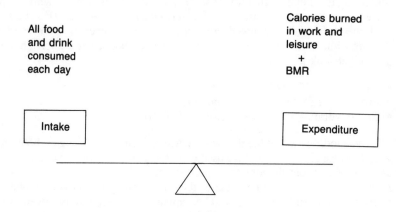

Figure 2. Relationship between energy intake and energy expenditure. If the total caloric intake equals the total energy expenditure, including the basal metabolic rate (BMR), then weight remains stable. If an imbalance is created, weight gain or loss results.

One final admonition for the athlete is to always maintain a hydrated body state. Research evidence indicates that a 3 to 5% loss of body weight by excessive sweating can reduce athletic performance. To ensure that this does not happen, the athlete must consume large amounts of water prior to and during the athletic event. The athlete can tell if they are well hydrated by having the urge to urinate frequently and voiding large amounts of mostly clear urine.

Summary

Good nutrition and optimal diet are necessary for topflight athletic competition. The well-prepared athlete is always well hydrated and consumes large amounts of good carbohydrates (whole grains, fruits, and fresh vegetables) in their diet. A suggested guideline is to allow 3 to 4 hours between eating and workouts.

Additional Reading

Morris, A.F. (1984). *Sports medicine: Prevention of athletic injuries*. Dubuque, IA: Wm. C. Brown.

The Basics of Wheelchair Selection and Positioning for Athletes With Cerebral Palsy

Ruth Burd

Kim Grass

Four major factors influence the performance of Class II through IV athletes. The main factor is the athlete. The individual's drive and determination, along with his or her self-image and natural ability, combine to make up performance. The athlete's training, wheelchair, and position in the wheelchair are the other factors.

When selecting an appropriate wheelchair, special consideration should be given to the wheels, rims, and the frame. Appendix C at the end of this book lists manufacturers.

Wheels

The power wheels normally used in athletic competition range from 24 in. to 700 cm and selection depends on the event. The 24-in. wheels are generally used in wheelchair soccer (Figure 1a) and slalom for quicker acceleration and greater maneuverability. Some athletes are experimenting with the use of smaller (20-in. or 22 in.) wheels for quicker directional changes in slalom (Figure 1b). For track

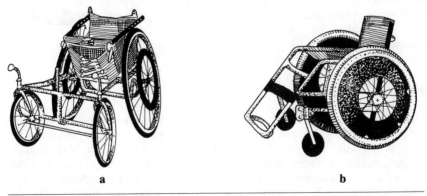

a   b

Figure 1. Modern racing track wheelchair (a) and slalom or wheelchair soccer (team handball) chair (b).

events, especially the races of Class II through IV athletes, the 700-cm wheels have the potential to roll at a faster pace. It is more difficult and requires greater strength to initiate movement of the larger wheels; however, once the movement begins, these wheels will allow greater speed (Figure 1a).

The tires should be high pressure pneumatics with pressures ranging from 45 to 60 PSI for the 24-in. tires of soccer and slalom chairs and 110 PSI for the 700-cm track tires. Sew-up tires are available that allow pressures up to 200 PSI. The higher pressures promote faster times. Quality hubs are considered top of the line and add the convenience of rapid wheel removal and wheel position changes.

Rims

Push rims vary in size and material. The appropriate rim size will depend on the strength and range of motion of the athlete. It takes more strength and greater mobility to push a wheelchair using 12-in. rims than it does using 18-in. rims. The 18-in. rims can lose their effectiveness as speed is gained. The athlete should be able to reach the rim in a position to maximize his or her forward propulsion and allow the longest possible stroke. The material covering the rim should be of a nonslip nature. For Class II lower extremity athletes, the rims add extra weight to the chair and should be removed.

For stability, the push wheels are cambered or tilted slightly inward, which brings the rims more directly under the athlete's shoulders. This allows the athlete to provide a straight vector of force to the wheel, thus using his or her available strength to its optimum level (Figure 4).

Spoke guards are available and prevent wheel damage from ramming. In addition, they also prevent injury to the athlete's hands. They are used primarily for wheelchair soccer.

The casters range from 4-in. hard nonpneumatic "basketball" wheels to a maximum of 18-in. pneumatic tires. For soccer and slalom, the 4-in. wheels are used to facilitate maneuverability. The casters should be adjusted by tightening them to prevent fluttering. For track, the pneumatic tires should be fully inflated, narrow, and have quality sealed bearings (Figure 1). Steering knobs are optional, depending upon the flexibility of the athlete. Many track chairs are equipped with caster tie rods that control their side-to-side movement and keep them parallel. In addition, crown compensators may be added to allow greater ease in steering on the track curves.

Frame

The frame of the wheelchair should be lightweight. Some materials currently used are stainless steel, which lasts longer and is more durable, aluminum, and titanium. Class II foot pushers frequently need additional weight to assist in chair control. A rigid, nonfolding frame is more stable and offers better alignment. With the larger casters, it is necessary to check their alignment frequently. Most commercially available chairs are provided with adjustable axle positions to allow for chair versatility. By changing the axle position, the chair can be used with a number of athletes. An adjustable seat back height is another option. Antitip extensions are important during soccer competition as a safety precaution.

Additional Considerations

The most critical criterion involving the performance of Class II through IV athletes is positioning in the wheelchair. This factor is important to consider before purchasing a sports wheelchair to be used solely for competition. The athlete and the coaching staff need to take the time to fully evaluate the competitor's disability specifically as it relates to his or her performance. Temporary modifications of the existing equipment can often be helpful in determining just what to look for in new equipment and may indicate the design of a custom chair.

In general terms, most persons classified as III and IV and having spastic involvement are extensor tone dominant. This means as they exert the necessary effort for athletic competition, they begin to lie in their chairs with their legs straightening out and coming off the footrests, hips popping off the seat, and shoulders pushing back. In addition, their stroke becomes extremely "choppy" and short, so that the front casters pop with each push. It is essential to break this extension pattern to allow maximal performance. This can be accomplished by purchasing a chair that has a built in "jackknife" seat; that is, a chair that has a less than 90° angle seat (Figure 2). For an athlete with an exceptionally strong extensor thrust, consider curving the top half of the seat-back forward. The chair width needs to be as narrow as possible without the athlete's hips rubbing against the wheels. As previously mentioned, this brings the wheels closer to the athlete and allows for a more direct push. If a custom chair is not available, adapt the existing equipment. Begin by strapping the athlete's ankles so that the knees remain bent and the feet are kept on the footrests. For some of the lesser involved athletes, this may be all that is necessary, but usually it will require adaptation of the seat position to keep the hips and trunk flexed as well. This is accomplished by using

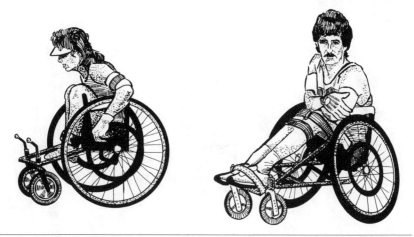

Figure 2. Two racing wheelchairs with difference degrees of angle in a "jackknife" seat.

a strap to make an elevated footrest so that the knees are higher than the hips. An additional strap coming from under the seat of the chair helps keep the person down and to the back of the seat, while also maintaining hip flexion. (Note: Refer to the article by Burd and Grass on strapping in this book for specifics.)

The Class II foot pusher presents some special characteristics that frequently necessitate the use of a custom designed wheelchair. For those Class II athletes who push going backward, it helps to have the caster wheels out of the way and reversed so that they lead the chair. These athletes usually turn to one side or the other to allow visualization of the course and to provide some additional stability (see Figure 3). It is useful to have the seat shifted specifically in this direction. A slight reverse angle (giving the seat a greater than 90° angle) allows greater use of the extensor tone. The seat depth should be the least possible but high enough so as not to interfere with the recover stroke.

For those Class II athletes who pull the chair with their feet, a more standard-looking chair is appropriate. Again the competitor needs to be positioned as far forward as possible to use the maximum excursion of his or her legs, but deep enough for adequate support. A seat belt at the hips is essential. The seat height will be higher than usual but is dependent on the person's leg length. Adjust the seat height to the highest height that allows continuous forward movement from a completely extended leg to a completely flexed leg without losing surface contact through the complete movement. The width should be as narrow as possible but the caster wheels must be spaced so as not to interfere with leg movement. This will necessitate a wider chair than otherwise used or a custom design. By using a rigid frame chair, the crossbar can be eliminated to allow a longer stride length. The seat would be firm, made of either tightly stretched material or a solid seat insert.

Specialized equipment may also be necessary for athletes who are extreme hemiplegics. In these situations, a standard wheelchair, whether it be a track chair or a slalom chair, is not particularly efficient. One-arm drive sports chairs are being seen more frequently, now that individualized custom wheelchairs are rapidly becoming the norm (see Figure 4). This recent technology has enabled many hemiplegics to be competitive in both track and slalom events.

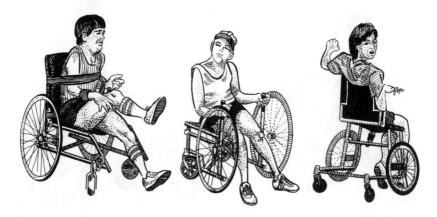

Figure 3. Various types of Class II lower wheelchairs.

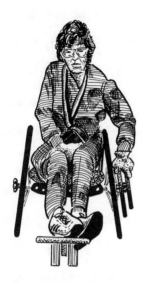 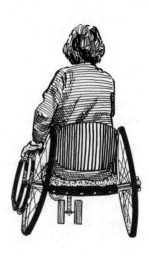

Figure 4. A one arm drive sports wheelchair for hemiplegic competition.

Conclusion

Although these guidelines are helpful, it is imperative to remember that positioning is an individual characteristic and each athlete should be fully evaluated by the coaching staff for possible changes in position or equipment to help improve function. Whenever possible, coaches should consult with the athlete's doctor and/or physical therapist. Watch the athlete push his or her existing equipment at different speeds, various distances, and through turns. Observe the difficulties encountered both in the movement patterns of the individual and in the chair design. From this evaluation, establish a list of possible alternatives that might help eliminate the problems. Begin by making modifications using pillows, straps, cushions, and cardboard inserts to the existing chair to establish the usefulness of the idea. Then make final adjustments before deciding on the design and purchase of a new wheelchair.

Additional Readings

Burk, C. (1986, March/April). Maximizing the positive. *Sport 'N Spokes,* pp. 12–16.

Crase, N. (1983, March/April). Survey of 1983 sport wheelchair manufacturers. *Sports 'N Spokes,* pp. 19–20.

Crase, N. (1984, March/April).The 1984 survey of sport wheelchair manufacturers. *Sports 'N Spokes.*

Crase, N. (1985, March/April). Survey of lightweight wheelchair manufacturers. *Sports 'N Spokes,* pp. 30–43.

Crase, N. (1986, March/April). 4th annual survey of the lightweights. *Sports 'N Spokes,* pp. 19–30.

Crase, N. (1986, March/April). Wheelchairs for juniors. *Sports 'N Spokes,* pp. 19–30.

Gibson, M., & Smith, W. (1983, March/April). The selection of sports wheelchairs. *Sports 'N Spokes,* pp. 25–28.

LaMere, T. & Labanowich, S. (1984, March/April). The history of sports wheelchairs—Part I. *Sports 'N Spokes,* pp. 6–11.

LaMere, T., & Labanowich, S. (1984, May/June). The history of sports wheelchairs—Part II. *Sports 'N Spokes,* pp. 12–15.

LaMere, T., & Labanowich, S. (1984, July/August). The history of sports wheelchairs—Part III. *Sports 'N Spokes,* pp. 12–16.

Rudwick, L. (1978, November/December). New equipment for wheelchair sports. *Sports 'N Spokes,* pp. 5–6.

Rudwick, L. (1979, November/December). Racing wheelchairs. *Sports 'N Spokes,* pp. 10–12.

Schuman, S. (1979, January/February). Wheelchair frame modifications. *Sports 'N Spokes,* pp. 5–6.

Spooren, P. (1981, November/December). The technical characteristics of wheelchair racing. *Sports 'N Spokes,* pp. 19–20.

The Use of Strapping to Enhance the Athletic Performance of Wheelchair Competitors in Cerebral Palsy Sports

Ruth Burd

Kim Grass

Proper positioning of an individual with cerebral palsy (CP) within a wheelchair is known to improve the everyday functional capabilities of that person. Proper positioning becomes even more important when that individual becomes involved in competitive or recreational sports. Although the athlete may use a variety of wheelchairs for different competitive events, the suggestions offered within this chapter will enhance his or her athletic performance regardless of the chair used.

The typical pattern of movement elicited in CP is the extension pattern characterized by hip, knee, and trunk extension, hip adduction and internal rotation, and ankle plantar flexion (toe pointing). This describes the position of an athlete who essentially ends up lying in his or her wheelchair when exerting maximal effort during competition (Figure 1a). In turn, the angle between the athlete and

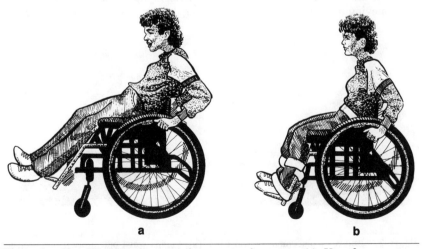

a   b

Figure 1. Class III athlete demonstrating an extension pattern (a). Use of proper strapping can diminish extension problems (b).

81

his or her wheel axle is increased, and the ability of the athlete to provide a full stroke on the handrim is decreased. In conjunction with wheelchair design, strapping can be used to diminish these problems (Figure 1b).

Evaluation of the athlete may reveal that controlling hip extension is sufficient to control the undesired pattern. A strap coming from under the chair will keep the athlete's hips secure in the chair. However, just wrapping a belt around the back of the chair will not keep the person from sliding forward under the strap as seen in Figure 2a. Proper strapping must come from under the seat at approximately a 45° angle and should be attached to the wheelchair frame as shown in Figure 2b. If affixed with the closure in the front, the athlete can fasten the strap to adjust the tension and is also able to free him- or herself in the event of a fall during competition.

Should the athlete's hips continue to extend, hip flexion may need to be increased. This can be accomplished by raising the footrests or by constructing a new foot support using a strap at a level higher than the footrest itself (Figure 3).

Frequently additional strapping will be necessary. You may find an athlete's feet pushing forward off the foot support even with a pelvic strap in place. A strap placed tightly across the front of the footrest from side to side will decrease the extension by keeping the knees in greater flexion. Placement of this strap should be as low as possible at the ankles.

In most United States Cerebral Palsy Athletic Association (USCPAA) wheelchair events, a strap behind the legs is already required for competition in order to prevent the feet from slipping off the back of the foot support. If not prevented, an athlete's feet may drag on the ground with hazardous results or become entangled in the casters. Allow a sufficient sag in this strap in order to properly position the feet on the footrest or elevated foot support. If the safety strap behind the legs is kept too tight, it will cause the feet to move too far forward It is also suggested that two separate straps be used to assure maintenance of proper position. If one long strap is used, it will slip so that it tightens behind the feet and loosens in front as the athlete pushes against it (see Figure 4).

For the athlete who is still thrusting or rotating in the wheelchair and therefore not achieving the best possible stroke, it may be necessary to provide straps to

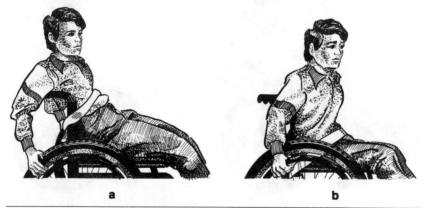

a   b

Figure 2.   Improper placement of waist belt (a), versus waist belt properly secured to frame, allowing correct positioning (b).

control the adduction component. Adduction in this case is pressing the thighs together. Frequently, the pull of one leg is stronger than the other, causing the athlete to rotate in the wheelchair seat, giving the appearance of being windswept.

Straps are placed around the thigh and tightened to the side frame of the wheelchair in order to pull the knees apart. One or both legs can be held in adduction, depending on the individual's position in the chair. If the right leg pulls in with forward rotation of the right hip, the right leg only would be strapped. If both legs are adducting, both legs are strapped.

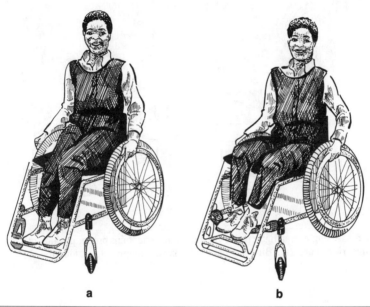

a   b

Figure 3.   Use of an additional strap raises footrest and allows for better flexion in knees and hips.

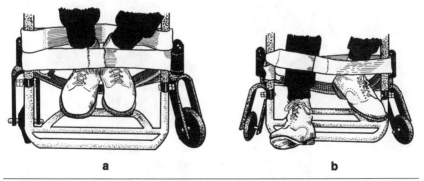

a   b

Figure 4.   A safety strap prevents legs from entanglement underneath wheelchair, a front strap helps to keep feet in proper position on footrest, and feet rest on an elevated footstrap (a). The use of one long strap may allow legs to slip through and off the footstrap (b).

An alternative technique for strapping to control hip adduction combined with internal rotation involves strapping the leg below the knees. Place the strap around the lower leg and fasten it to the upright of the foot support (see Figure 5). Caution should be taken when using this option. One should evaluate the athlete's knees for medial-lateral stability prior to using this technique.

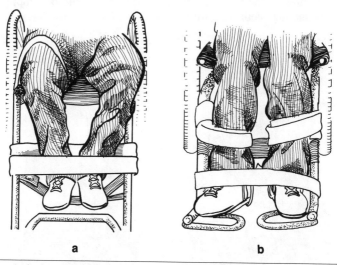

a   b

Figure 5.   A single strap tightened to the side frame maintains proper position of a stronger adducting right knee (a). Bilateral below-the-knee strapping for adduction (b).

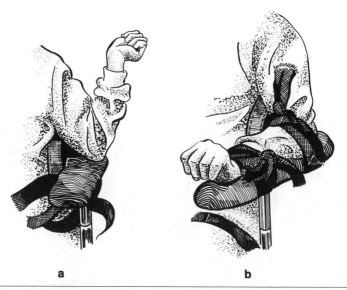

a   b

Figure 6.   Left arm prior to strapping (a). The use of two straps secures the forearm in a neutral position (b).

Due to increased flexion, an athlete's ankles may dorsiflex so that his or her toes lift off the foot support. A strap attached to the footrest can be placed over the feet to press the feet down onto the foot support.

For Class I one-arm drive and Class II lower athletes, strapping of one or more upper extremities may be necessary. The principle is the same. Use your straps to achieve optimal positioning for function and to inhibit unwanted patterns of movement. For example, to control spastic patterns and athetoid movements in the upper extremities, strap the forearm to the armrest in a neutral position, as seen in Figure 6. The straps can be attached permanently using the existing screws of the armrest, or if the sports chair being used does not have armrests, the frame of the chair can be used.

Due to the variability of upper extremity patterns, it is suggested that you consult with a physical or occupational therapist experienced in concepts of positioning prior to initiating any upper extremity strapping. This may also be necessary if extreme difficulty is encountered when properly positioning an athlete.

General Precautions

When using straps, it is important to be aware of any areas of decreased sensation (which is rare in CP) that could be prone to skin breakdowns. All strapped areas should be checked for redness. Straps should be made of wide 2-in. webbing to reduce the chance of irritation. Velcro fasteners or buckles allow frequent adjustment and quick release.

Be aware of color changes or swelling following strapping. If an athlete complains of unusual sensations, it is time to loosen and adjust the straps. This could indicate placement of the strap is over a nerve or blood vessel. As a general rule, all straps should be loosened when not in competition or active practice, especially those around the extremities.

Part III

Specific Activities

Training Techniques for Track Events

Janice Tetreault
Paul Tetreault

For any athlete to be successful in track competition, he or she must engage in a program of progressive exercise and endurance training.[1] One should be aware of certain principles when dealing with track competition. The first and perhaps the most important commandment of running and/or wheeling is "train, don't strain." When embarking on a proper training program, one should strive to obtain a good general physical condition.

Flexibility and loose muscle action are vital to success; thus a proper warm-up and cool-down are very important. All runners, whether they are sprinters or distance runners, should also develop a solid long-distance base. This will provide the athlete with a firm foundation upon which speed and stamina can be built. As the season progresses, the athlete gradually develops into speed work, always moving with control of the body. Caution must be used with speed workouts. Too much emphasis on speed alone yields injury and/or staleness. Speed workouts should be avoided during cold weather, unless you have access to an indoor track. Develop upper and lower body strength to their optimum. Many times it is the use of the arms that provides the balance and explosive power needed for a finishing kick. When running or wheeling, always think about relaxing and moving with correct form. Remember—a flexible muscle will be a strong muscle. In track, wheelchair and foot racing are thought of as one for this article, except where noted.

It is also important for a coach/trainer to create a positive enjoyable atmosphere. One should remember to:

1. Set realistic goals and objectives.
2. Discipline—be consistently firm but fair.
3. Know your athlete's abilities. This aids in planning efficient training sessions to reach your athlete's goals.
4. Evaluate and reward progress. Evaluation can be in the form of observations, time improvements, attitude assessment; rewards can be in the form of praise, medals, or a pat on the back.

As a coach/trainer it is imperative that you earn the respect of your athletes by being knowledgeable about your sport, consistent, realistic, sensitive to the needs of your athletes, flexible, motivating, confident, and assertive.

Warm-Ups and Cool-Downs

Flexibility of muscles is vital for success in track events, so before running or conditioning exercises, the body should be warmed up to increase respiration and body temperature and to stretch ligaments and connective tissue. Preworkout or premeet warm-up should include calisthenics and flexibility exercises (see Figure 1). Some suggestions include the following exercises:

- *Wall push-up or calf stretcher*—Stand in front of wall, extend arms forward and touch wall with fingertips. Keep the heels flat on the floor throughout the exercise; bend arms and touch chest to the wall.
- *Arm circles*—Extend arms sideways at shoulder height, palms up. Move arms in small circles and gradually progress to large circles. Reverse direction.
- *Trunk twist*—Twist the trunk of your body from side to side.
- *Bent-leg sit-ups*—Sit up, rolling shoulders off floor the length of spine, keeping knees bent.
- *Leg raises*—Lie on your back with your right knee flexed, foot on the floor, and your left leg straight. Slowly raise your left leg until it points straight up. Lower your left leg and repeat the whole sequence with the right leg.
- *Push-ups*—Keeping the legs straight on toes, extend arms and push body up keeping the legs straight. In a wheelchair you can push up into a straight-arm support on chair arms.
- Walking, jogging, or wheeling.

Proper stretching before and after vigorous exercise will decrease stiffness and fatigue and prevent injuries. Refer to the chapter by Rusling in this book for more specifics on flexibility exercises.

Basic Principles of Coaching

Establish *season goals* and *intermediate objectives* for every event in which an individual athlete participates. Such direction provides a basis for determining pacing and training times for workouts and practice sessions. Intermediate objectives are established according to scheduled times that key meets are held through-

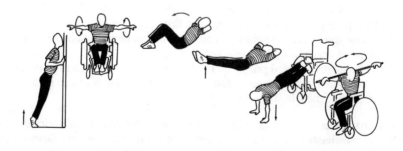

Figure 1.   Various stretching and calisthenics exercises.

out the competitive seasons. Both season goals and intermediate objectives must be periodically reviewed and adjusted (faster or slower) in terms of times in actual competition and progress during training workouts and practice sessions. Goals and objectives must be designed to challenge the individual athlete, make him or her reach and stretch, and bring out every ability.

Keep a personal log that includes (a) warm-up activities and how each specific activity and combination makes the individual feel, (b) season goals and intermediate objectives, (c) information about training workouts and practice sessions, (d) pace splits from competition, (e) times from training workouts and practice sessions, (f) information about opponents, and (g) any other information about conditions to help the athlete perform better and more effectively.

Experiment with different warm-up patterns and approaches until the best and most appropriate one for the individual athlete is determined. Continue to experiment with slight modifications in warm-up procedures so that they become even better and more effective for the individual.

Determine how warm-up patterns and approaches differ for practice and competition in terms of specific activities, repetitions, and timing. Practice warm-up routines include stretching and flexibility exercises as well as strength and endurance activities, form work, and emphasis on the special needs of each athlete. Premeet warm-up routines and approaches include few if any strength and endurance activities and place more emphasis on preparing for actual competitive events.

Training tips for coaches include the following:

- Include weight training or resistance training as both an off and regular season supplement to basic training in track.
- Plan workouts so each athlete's primary competitive distance is only done in actual competition—save these efforts for meets; don't leave championship performances in practice!
- Emphasize quantity of work during pre- and early season; gradually give more attention to quality of work in mid- and late season.
- Good running/wheeling is an accumulation of much running/wheeling. Correct practice does make perfect.

Types of Training

The first time you train, don't plan to go far. The most important aspect of an athlete's training is consistency. He must make exercising a healthy habit and train a minimum of 4 days per week. There are various types of programs:

- *Walk-wheel-jog-run*—This applies to the initial conditioning of an athlete. The athlete can start with doing the warm-up exercises and then walking (wheeling) to jogging for short distances and finally cooling down for recovery. As one's condition improves, so should the distance covered increase. It is important to work up to the point of being able to cover a somewhat demanding amount of distance so as to build the foundation for the various methods of speed training to follow.

- *Interval workouts*—Used for various purposes—speed strength, endurance, pace, and rhythm. Intervals are timed on a track or over an exactly measured course. Four important factors involving interval workouts: (a) distance to be timed, (b) pace distance to be covered, (c) number of repetitions, and (d) time between reps.
- *Fartlek*—This is a Swedish word meaning "speed play." In it you perform a series of fast untimed runs over a variety of distances and terrains. It is a workout that is hard work, yet can be fun. This method avoids the monotony and repetition encountered with track workouts. For example, you might devise a 2-mile route that includes flat straightaways, a couple of rolling hills, a field to cross, and so on. You decide the points where you will push hard, and where you will alternate with a slower pace.
- *Pace workouts*—These workouts are vital for developing an athlete's internal stopwatch. Try to run a component part of your race distance at a slightly faster pace for a predetermined number of repetitions. Rule of thumb: Even pace is the most economical and effective approach.
- *Speed work*—Speed is important for fast starts, fighting off challenges, and fast finishes. Several types of speed workouts include:
  (1) Wind sprints—sprint full speed various short distances while maintaining maximum relaxation
  (2) Ins and outs—spring curves (ins) and move easily the straightaways (outs)
  (3) Relays—continuous laps with small groups. This controls a rest/work cycle.
- *Hill or ramp work*—Hill workouts are an important training tool for competitors of all distances. A hill or ramp approximately 20 to 30 meters long with a gradual slope is ideal. On one day, work the downhill (especially good for sprinters). On another day, work the uphill portion by going up fast and coasting back down for a specific number of repetitions or period of time. On the downhills, athletes wheel as fast as possible with control. This allows an athlete to move faster than normal sprinting and trains arm and leg muscles in speedier responses and reactions. This should also be done for a specific number of repetitions or period of time.

Starting

Good starting mechanics can make the difference between victory and defeat. Practice starting form and work to have each athlete in a position with their center of gravity as far forward as possible (see Figure 2). Use "reaction starts" where an athlete develops reactions to *sound* of any type and vary the cadence of the starting commands. Do starting drills at full speed. Before competition season, get the athlete conditioned to the type of start (i.e., gun, flag, or whistle) that he or she will have to face in competition.

Finishing

Many races are won not by the athlete who can accelerate fastest but by those who slow down the least. A race is not over until a competitor is across the finish line. Encourage athletes to run or wheel beyond the finish line and an additional

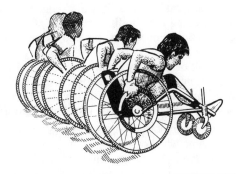

Figure 2. Class IV athletes practicing starts.

10 m to ensure an all-out finish and to reduce the chance of injury through sudden stops.

When planning your program, plan it around the "hard day/easy day" principle. A strenuous workout one day should be followed by an easy workout the following day. Don't expect quick results. If you try to do too much too soon, you are inviting injury. Improvement will eventually take place.

Techniques

Now that we have an idea on how to begin and what to do to devise a training program, we should constantly review the running or wheeling technique.

Head. When running/wheeling, one should focus his eyes approximately 12 to 15 yd ahead. You should try to relax your facial muscles; that is, don't squint your eyes or wrinkle your brow. This will reserve your energy for the movement. Look straight ahead and avoid the swaying head effort. Try to breathe naturally through the nose and mouth.

Arms. (Running). Your arms should swing from the shoulders. For distance runners, the arms' most important responsibility is to help maintain momentum and balance. They should be held low around waist height and as relaxed as possible. Hands should be gently cupped to help arms relax. Sprinters use their arms to assist with the explosive power needed for sustained performances. When sprinting, arms should swing in a vigorous alternating motion from the shoulders and be held slightly higher than waist height.

(Wheelchairs) The most effective technique, which is circular in motion, requires a specific wheelchair structure and especially a specific size of handrims. To maintain maximum pushing efficiency, the duration of the arms' push phase must be as long as possible. The recovery phase must be kept as short as possible. The arms should make a revolving, circular motion with the hands in which the grip on the handrims is only loosened to allow repositioning. Push forward with the hand if followed by a backward pull on the rim.

Handrim size is determined by the range of motion, strength of the athlete, and the distance of the race (i.e., usually the longer the distance of the race, the smaller the hand rim).

Trunk. (Running). The trunk of the body will change the angle of its lean depending on the distance being run. In distance racing, the body should be held in a relaxed, upright position. For sprints, the body should assume a slight forward lean.

(Wheelchair) The trunk of the body should lean forward in the chair to help assist in a smooth rhythmic pull. By bending the trunk forward at the hips or by bringing the knees up to a higher level that will cause a more pronounced sitting angle, the pushing movement will be less downward and more forward.

Legs. The legs play a very important part of a successful training program. The basic concepts are the same whether you use your legs to run or to propel your wheelchair. The shorter the distance, the longer the stride. You always want to start running with the muscles properly stretched and warmed up so as to prevent injury. You do not want to take very long strides or you risk the danger of tying up and slowing down.

Race Strategy

Race strategy is very important in being a successful track athlete. Not always does the swiftest runner win, but often victory goes to the smarter competitor. Know your fellow opponents and try to assess their strengths and weaknesses. If your opponent appears to possess a faster finishing kick, then you should try to force him or her to extend that speed over the long haul and thus minimize the kick.

When starting, always put your stronger foot forward so as to get a strong initial push-off. Follow this with a rhythmic pace that you can hold during the majority of races. You must exercise control and run within your limits. When running in a short straightaway race, you must always stay in your lane, but for the longer races, you should cut into the inside lane once a substantial lead is obtained over the nearest rival. Never look back while running; every time you do this, you lose a half step and inform your opponent of your being tired. Never slow up before the finish line; always run through the finish line and gradually slow your pace down to a stop.

Equipment

If you are going to be an athlete, you should look the part. One of the advantages of track racing is the rather inexpensive cost of equipment. For those running or wheeling you should wear a pair of running shorts, T-shirt, clean white socks, warm-up suit, and running shoes. Wheelchair competitors also may want to experiment with using leather golf gloves to help prevent blisters.

Note

Individuals interested in obtaining a copy of the able-bodied track event rules as well as training and coaching texts on track events should contact: The Athletic Congress of the USA, 200 South Capitol Avenue, Suite 140, Indianapolis, IN 46225, (317) 638-9155

Additional Readings

Cooper, K. (1970). *The new aerobics*. NY: Bantam Books.

Doherty, K.J. (1963). *Modern track and field*. Englewood Cliffs, NJ: Prentice-Hall.

Emmerton, B. (1978). *The official book of running*. NY: Book Craft Guild.

Fixx, J. (1977). *The complete book of running*. NY: Random House.

Henderson, J. (1977). *Jog, run, race*. Mountain View, CA: World Publication.

The Runner. NY: Ziff-Davies.

Runner's World Magazine. World Publications.

Spooren, P. (1981, December). The technical characteristics of wheelchair racing. *Sports 'N Spokes*.

General Considerations for Field Events

Jeffery A. Jones

The area of field events is the single most diversified area of sports found within the cerebral palsy (CP) sport umbrella. The 11 different events offered under the auspices of the United States Cerebral Palsy Athletic Association (USCPAA) and the classes that participate in each are listed in Table 1.

Writing a single chapter on all 11 events is almost as difficult as coaching all of them. What I will attempt to do in this chapter is introduce you to a variety of common issues that should be considered when coaching field events. What I will not be doing is repeating what has already been discussed in other chapters in terms of warming up, flexibility, proper positioning in a wheelchair, and weight training. Coaches and athletes should refer to those other chapters for specific information pertaining to field events.

Because most individuals interested in coaching field events are already familiar with the four common field events (shotput, discus, javelin, and long jump) and because volumes of material are already available in respect to coaching these events, the majority of my discussion will be specific to those events unique to USCPAA competition. However, initially I would like to discuss several factors applicable to all field events.

Table 1 USCPAA Field Events

Class I	High toss, distance throw, precision throw, soft discus
Class II (Lower)	Thrust kick, distance kick
Class II (Upper)	Club, shot, discus
Class III	Club, shot, discus
Class IV	Club, shot, discus, javelin
Class V	Club, shot, discus, javelin
Class VI	Club, shot, discus, javelin
Class VII	Shot, discus, javelin, long jump
Class VIII	Shot, discus, javelin, long jump

Technique

The Able-Bodied Way

For the events that apply, coaches are advised to have a good understanding of able-bodied techniques. Hundreds of books are available on the subject. Many of these include frame-by-frame photographic breakdowns of athletes' throwing styles and techniques. Hundreds of years of practice, coupled with modern technology, have provided able-bodied athletes with the most efficient ways to accomplish a given athletic task. Depending on the event and the athlete, the use of able-bodied techniques may or may not be appropriate. What an able-bodied athlete does with his legs in the shotput will have little to do with a Class III or IV shotputter (see Figure 1). However, the action and angle of the putting arm, along with the rotation of the upper body, certainly will.

Able-bodied techniques will, of course, play a bigger part in coaching the ambulatory athlete. Whenever possible, ambulatory athletes should attempt to learn specific able-bodied techniques. Balance and coordination may be the two biggest factors preventing success. However, patience and a great deal of practice usually overcome balance and coordination, given time.

There may also be difficulties with an athlete's ability to acquire a given motor skill. One must remember that cerebral palsy connotes some type of motor dysfunction. In many cases, individuals with CP have not been afforded the same benefits of good elementary and secondary physical education as their able-bodied counterparts. Many of the motor skills and motor patterns taught to and learned by able-bodied children are often absent in children with disabilities. This may be particularly true for wheelchair athletes. A recent study done at the University of Connecticut (Roper, 1985) cited finding a number of "immature throwing patterns." The study also stated that "an apparent lack of instruction which would enable transition from this immature pattern to a mature pattern appears to be the reason for a lag in development by many of this population."

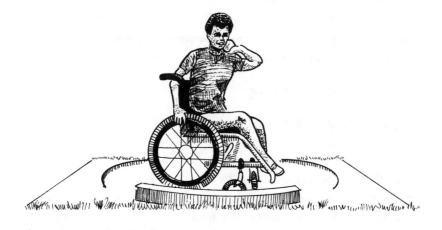

Figure 1. Class III shot putter.

Many coaches often instruct through *passive movement* in order to overcome an athlete's difficulty in learning a particular skill. This method of teaching involves physically moving the athlete through a sequence of movements so that the athlete can physically feel and visually see what the coach is expecting them to do (see Figure 2). After a period of time, this may help an athlete develop a kinesthetic and tactile awareness of how his or her body should feel when properly performing a skill.

Another teaching method commonly used by coaches is the "whole-part method." This teaching style suggests that most activities can and should be broken down into small, simple parts. Each part is learned separately in a development sequence until the entire skill or task is acquired. Coaches are cautioned not to move an athlete along too quickly. Fundamental motor skills should be learned completely and accurately before proceeding to the next level of skill acquisition.

There Is No Right Way

After 8 years of coaching CP athletes, the most important thing I've learned is there is no right way to do anything. This is most certainly the case in the area of field events. Although the majority of athletes will perform with the conventional overhand and underhand throwing motions, there will be those who will not. There are a variety of factors including spasticity, reduced range of motion, uneven muscle strength, and balance that will prevent an athlete from using conventional throwing motions. At times, coaches need to look past able-bodied techniques

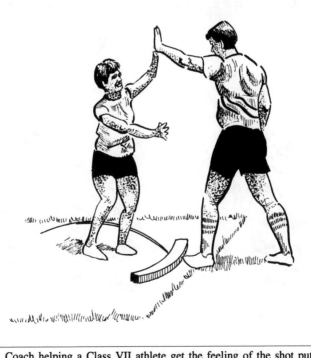

Figure 2.   Coach helping a Class VII athlete get the feeling of the shot put.

and fully evaluate their athletes' abilities. This thought is simply depicted in Figure 3. The athlete who, because of upper extremity spasticity and reduced range of movement (ROM), found it more efficient to use an across-the-chest abduction motion rather than an overhand or underhand motion (Figure 3a). In Figure 3b, another nonconventional technique is demonstrated. In both cases, successful methods are based on the athlete's own ability, not standard or expected able-bodied techniques.

There will be no correct way to do any single event. Considering all the different classes you have to work with, combined with the variety of abilities within each class, a coach needs to be flexible in his or her approach toward field event techniques.

Momentum: The Few Extra Inches

Momentum, speed, and power are all essential factors for successful field event performances. Too often coaches forget the importance of these factors when working with CP athletes.

Spins, glides, and approach runs are all used by able-bodied athletes to generate the necessary momentum and power to produce the optimal performance. The difficulties with balance and coordination discussed earlier often prevent the CP athlete from using these techniques. Coaches and athletes need to understand that it is not an all or nothing situation. If your Class VII discus thrower is unable to complete the two rotation discus spin, do not altogether dismiss the possibility of using a spin. The athlete may be able to perform a one rotation or three quarters

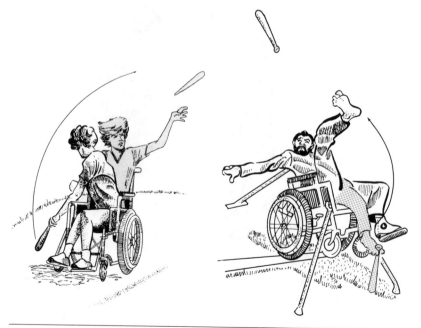

Figure 3.   Alternatives to conventional throwing motions in the clubthrow.

of a rotation spin with time and practice. Again, the importance is to evaluate the athlete's abilities and to compensate for those not present. Too many Class VI, VII, and VIII athletes don't use proper technique for the easy reason, "I can't do that." Coaches need to impress upon these athletes that they are giving away valuable inches (even feet) by not using momentum-producing techniques. The time spent practicing can often make the difference.

This discussion also applies to wheelchair athletes. Too often wheelchair athletes throw without the power and momentum created by upper body rotation. In most cases, athletes, regardless of the class, should be able to create some additional momentum by involving their hips, trunk, shoulders, and head into the throwing motion (see Figure 4). Using a wheelchair with a lower back, which allows greater trunk rotation, more specific use of the nonthrowing arm and stabilization of the athlete's wheelchair during the throw may all result in a better overall performance.

Whether it be a Class V athlete needing a crutch for balance, a Class IV shot-putter, or a Class VIII javelin thrower, coaches should closely consider and experiment with and incorporate into their athletes' throwing styles as much momentum-creating techniques as possible.

Wasted Motion/Wasted Energy

Have you ever watched an athlete take 10 warm-up swings and then have a bad throw? This phenomenon, most often seen in the discus and club throw events, is a bad habit developed by many athletes and should not be confused with proper momentum-creating techniques. I try to have my athletes develop a simple routine in order to break this habit. Prior to entering the throwing area, I have them make a mental picture of what they are about to do, concentrating specifically on all those good habits and techniques they worked on in practice and actually visualize themselves performing the throw. They run through it once or twice in their minds and then physically do it—short and sweet. No enormous amount of energy is wasted on 10 or so warm-up swings, just two or three with everything

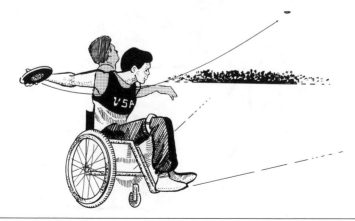

Figure 4. Class IV discus thrower using good upper body rotation in order to produce extra momentum.

concentrated on the final explosive motion. This should be part of an athlete's daily practice so that everything becomes an automatic part of his or her competitive routine.

Practice Without Practicing: The Prevention of Burnout

One of the most frustrating things facing the CP athlete is lack of competition. In many parts of the country there may be only one official competition per year. This leaves a considerable amount of time to practice too much of some things and not enough of other things.

Athletes need to spend more time on fundamentals and technique and less time throwing implements. Too many athletes start throwing all out too early in the season and wind up either injured or burnt out midway through the spring. One of the best things a coach can do early in a season is to leave the field implements out of sight and out of mind (see Figure 5).

There are a number of developmental training activities including flexibility, weight training, and technique work that athletes could be doing instead of throwing out their arms 6 months before their only competition. Coaches should spend time teaching all the basics of competition. Proper precompetition warm-up, entering, positioning and leaving the circle, knowledge and understanding of rules, and behavior toward officials and other competitors are all as important to the final product as the ability to throw. All should be a part of your regular practice. Bad habits are easily learned and very hard to break. Spend the time early doing the right things. There will always be plenty of time to throw.

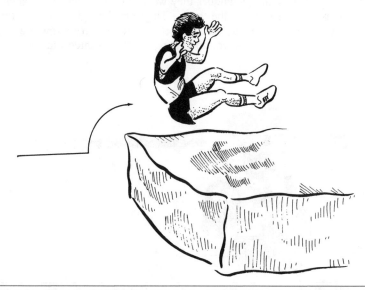

Figure 5. The use of a high jump mat for practicing long jump landings in preseason help save the legs for competition.

There are also a number of ways to break up the monotony of the long season of practice after practice. Many coaches use intersquad practice meets to help prepare athletes both physically and mentally for the real thing. Also, an unexpected change in routine, like a surprise wheelchair team handball game or a free night of swimming provides a good workout while also changing the pace of your everyday workout.

Class I Events

The following throwing events are appropriate for Class I athletes:

- *Distance throw*—As the name implies, the distance throw involves throwing an implement, the soft shot, as far as possible.
- *Soft discus*—Similar to the conventional discus event, a round implement (such as a cloth flippy flyer) is thrown for distance.
- *Precision event*—The athlete participating in the precision event attempts to accumulate the highest possible score by means of six throws at a large target with eight consecutive rings (see Figure 6).
- *High toss*—The high toss is the newest Class I event incorporated by USCPAA (see Figure 7). It involves throwing a soft shot over a progressively higher

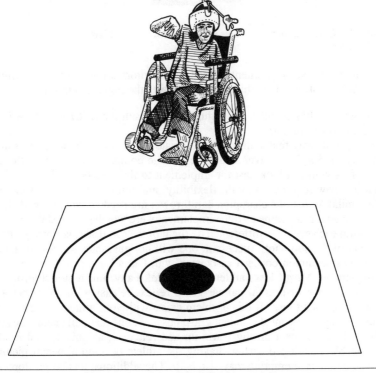

Figure 6. A Class I athlete using a head stick in the precision event.

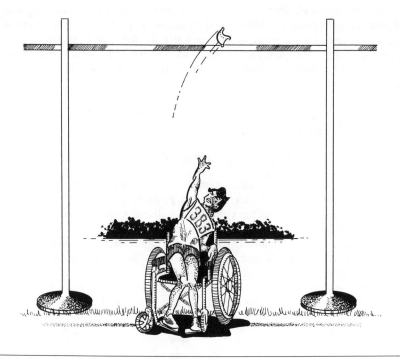

Figure 7.   Class I athlete uses an overhead throw in the high toss.

bar. Pole vault equipment is used, competitors are given three attempts at each height, and the athlete throwing over the highest height is the winner.

For more specifics on rules and regulations, consult the *USCPAA Classification and Sport Rules Manual*.

Some people may find it difficult to associate such field implements as a soft shot (beanbag) and a flippy flyer with true athletic competition. Luckily, there are those of us who can look past the implement to the skill being developed. The distance throw requires strength, flexibility, and timing. In the precision event, skills similar to that of a champion dart thrower are needed, whereas with the soft discus the goal is the same as if the implement were wooden. The skills necessary to perform each event are different. The flight of the soft discus is entirely different than that of the soft shot. Success in one will not guarantee success in another.

The most common concern associated with Class I athletes is the release of the implement. Most Class I athletes have little, if any, fine motor control. Combined with the ever-present palmar grasp reflex, releasing an object can be an extremely difficult task. If this problem exists with your athlete, time should be spent developing the most efficient grasp possible; one that will enable the athlete to hold the implement during warm-up and release it as quickly and easily as possible. As mentioned earlier, having the athlete develop a mental picture of what he or she is attempting may also help. The additional mental reinforcement may help connect the thoughts of the brain with the actions of the arm, hand,

and fingers. Time spent on just the release, just simply letting go of the implement without concentrating on the throwing motion, may also help.

Coaches are reminded that conventional overhanded and underhanded throwing motions may not be practical for your Class I athlete. However, as with other classes, there are alternatives. Experiment. Come up with the most efficient grasp and throwing motion possible. As in most events, consistency is important; patience and practice are the keys.

Class II Foot Events

As in the Class I events, Class II foot kicking events are unique to CP sports. In the early stages of development, it was thought important that appropriate field events be found for athletes with lower extremity dominance. The thrust and distance kick were the answer.

With the exception of two major rules, the events are very similar. In terms of implements, the thrust kick uses a 6-lb medicine ball whereas a 13-in. rubber utility ball is used in the distance kick. The second difference is in regard to rules. In the thrust kick, the athlete's foot must maintain contact with the ball at all times prior to the kick. In the distance kick, the athlete is not required to maintain contact (see Figure 8). This rule difference provides the athlete with the opportunity to wind up prior to kicking the ball.

The majority of Class II athletes will use a straight-on kicking style for both the thrust and distance kick. There are some, however, that find that they can create a more powerful kick through a lateral adducting motion using the inside of the foot.

Some of your kickers will have an extreme extensor thrust reflex. Any attempt to forcefully extend the leg will produce an almost immediate contraction of the hamstrings, thus preventing full extension of the lower leg. If this reflex is present, you should spend time experimenting with varied kicking speeds. Try to determine which speed produces the fullest extension and/or best kick.

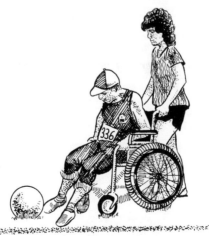

Figure 8.   Class II athlete uses a side kick motion in the distance kick.

Consistency is important. Ball placement and foot position should be worked on extensively. Find that point that provides maximum kicking power. While kicking, your athlete may have difficulty positioning the nonkicking leg so that it does not interfere with the movement of the ball. A simple solution is to tuck the foot around the back of the caster wheel. If the athlete has difficulty keeping the leg out of the way during the entire kick, it may be necessary to strap the leg down. Caution should be taken whenever strapping is used.

Experience Can Help Even the Best Teacher

I was only able to discuss a portion of what is important to field event coaches. My best advice is to try it yourself. It's difficult to teach horseback riding without ever being on a horse, or archery without ever shooting an arrow. Take the time. Grab a wheelchair and some field implements and develop an appreciation and feel for what you are trying to teach to someone else. If you or your coaching staff is not familiar with a particular event, seek outside assistance. More and more high school and college coaches of able-bodied sports are becoming involved in disabled sports programs. Many are just waiting to be asked.

My final suggestion will be to never lose your creativity. Whether it be using videotape playback as a teaching tool, entering your athlete into a local able-bodied track and field competition, or registering your team as members of The Athletic Congress of the United States (TAC), our job as coaches is to provide our athletes with as many positive learning experiences as possible. The experiences are out there for the choosing. All we have to do is decide to take advantage of them.

Note

Individuals interested in obtaining a copy of the able-bodied Field Event Rules, as well as training and coaching texts on field events should contact: The Athletic Congress of the USA, 200 South Capitol Avenue, Suite 140, Indianapolis, IN 46225, (317) 638-9155

Reference

Roper, P. (1985). *Throwing patterns of athletes with cerebral palsy Classes I-IV*. Unpublished manuscript.

Coaching the Slalom

Jerry Lewis

The slalom is an event where the mind, the body, and the equipment must work as one. This development of integrated harmony among the parts is what both the athlete and coach strive for. A successful athlete can be measured by how well the coach meshes the parts into a whole by maximizing the athlete's areas of strength and minimizing the areas of weakness.

This is no easy task to undertake, for it will require many hours of hard work on the part of the athlete and coach to find the correct formula for success. This is because success is not an overnight occurrence but is a process that develops over time, with success being the final outcome.

The process begins with an assessment of each individual athlete from which specialized training programs will be developed. Some of the areas to be considered in such an assessment include equipment, positioning, and individual athletic ability.

Equipment

How well suited is your athlete's present wheelchair to the specific needs of the Slalom? Specifically, you should consider the following points (see Figure 1):

- Is the wheelchair the proper weight? If too heavy, it can add on needless additional seconds. If too light it can create severe control problems, adding senseless errors, and causing added time.

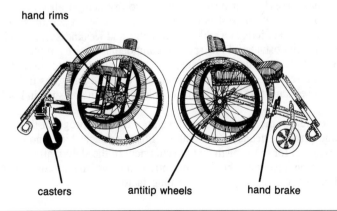

Figure 1. Wheelchair equipped for the slalom.

- Are the hand rims too big or too small for your athlete? Either way they can reduce the efficiency of the athlete's push so that needless power is wasted. Are the hand rims too slippery or too sticky? This also can create control problems resulting in wasted seconds. Would racing gloves help or hinder the performance?
- Are the antitip wheels up or down? What is the best position for them to facilitate a successful run?
- Are the casters the proper size, and should they be rubberized or air filled? The correct combinations can decrease final times substantially.
- Is the athlete presently practicing the slalom with hand brakes still in the original position? If so, this can not only possibly injure the athlete but can, at times and unknowingly, become engaged, causing an accident, or simply slowing down times.

Positioning

The athlete should be positioned in such a way that his posture promotes increased pushing power and control, along with improved visual acuity for timing and accuracy. Coaches need to promote the proper use of strapping and belting to its full advantage. When used correctly, the athlete benefits greatly from increased stability. When possible, coaches should consult with a physical therapist for recommendations. For more information, refer to the section of this manual on positioning and wheelchair selection.

Individual Athletic Ability

The slalom requires the combination of speed and agility through a series of four obstacles: (a) one 360° circle, (b) one 360° gate and three reverse gates, (c) one figure eight, and (d) one ramp (see Figure 2).

A coach's job will be to determine what obstacles create the most problems for your athlete and why. What simple yet specific solutions can be devised to circumvent the weaknesses? What obstacles create no problem at all when being run through and why? Can these strengths be applied to correct certain weaknesses? In order to accurately judge an athlete's strengths and weaknesses, a coach should break down each obstacle into its specific components. For example, the reverse gate, most difficult of the four obstacles, can be divided into three parts—the approach, the reverse, and the exit. Each one of these parts has unique movements unto itself, and this enables you to isolate problem areas for individualized work.

The next step in the process is to develop a training program that meets the mental and physical needs of the athlete. For the coach this is no easy chore, but it is essential for the growth and development of the slalom athlete. A proper overall training program should concentrate on two major components—the motivation factor and the physical training factor.

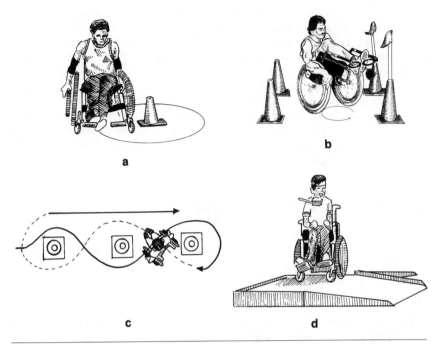

Figure 2.   The four components of the slalom course: (a) one 360° circle, (b) one 360° gate and three reverse gates, (c) one figure eight, and (d) one ramp.

Motivation Factor

There are two types of motivation that coaches should be concerned with, extrinsic and intrinsic.

The *extrinsic* type of motivation is the one the coach can control and manipulate to the athlete's advantage in workouts. Here, by constantly changing the training environment, you are not allowing the athlete to become lulled into boredom. Allowed to seep into your program, boredom can destroy the athlete's ability to reach his potential and eternally frustrate the coach. Coaches should consider some very basic ideas that have extrinsic motivational factors built in when developing an athlete's practice schedule. Do not be afraid to have fun with your practices. It will be easier for your athletes to work hard if they enjoy what they are doing. Vary your drills. The same skill activity can be approached in a multitude of ways. This not only broadens the variety of workouts you can offer, but it also prevents your athlete from getting tunnel vision or the perception that there is only one way to do a particular skill. Finally, coaches should always build into the program an occasional recreation night. Let your athletes know that you appreciate their hard work and that it will be rewarded as the year goes on.

The other type of motivation you hope to foster within your athlete is referred to as *intrinsic*. This is not as easily controlled by the coach as the extrinsic type. Here, you must try to develop within the athlete a feeling of self-worth or drive. Once you are able to tap those resources, the performance level can only escalate.

Coaches should remember to teach and explain the reasons behind specific work regimens and skill training, and how it affects them. A well-informed athlete is a hard-working and smart individual, a coach's delight.

Also, coaches should set aside time for a slalom team meeting every other practice or so. Let each athlete know that you see them not only as athletes but as individuals as well. This will allow them to grow individually and as important members of a group.

The Physical Training Factor

There is little doubt that in order to be successful in slalom, an athlete must concentrate heavily on proper training. The event requires strength, speed, and agility. Coaches should address each of them individually.

Strength

When competing in the slalom, there are three critical points where strength or power play a pivotal role: pulling out of the reverse gate, pushing up the ramp, and reaching down for the "little extra" needed for the final sprint to the finish. These areas must have specialized drills so that the specific muscle groups involved are exercised to their fullest in a very functional manner.

Speed

When measured, the slalom course is approximately 70 m long. This distance in itself identifies the slalom as a sprinter's event. So, a modified sprinter's workout should be included in the training schedule. Areas of concentration should be the start, the finish, and work in proper body alignment.

Agility

Built into the slalom are 17 directional changes for athletes to contend with. The ability of your athlete to effectively handle and deal with these changes of direction is paramount for a successful run. Specific drills must be incorporated into workouts to meet this need. Because most athletes will be interested in other events, slalom practice can be easily integrated into a weekly workout schedule.

Sample Training Program

The following is an example of a possible training program that can run in three parts for a 10-month period (September to June), twice a week for 45 minutes.

Part I.   Off-Season Training (September to November)

A. 25 minutes—Strength/Sprinter Speed/Agility Drills
- *Strength* Weight pushes—pushing weighted-down wheelchair
  5 m pullback—propelling wheelchair in reverse direction
- *Speed* 30 m sprints
  Starts, finishes, body positioning
- *Agility* 15 seconds of directional changes on command

B. 15 minutes—Individual Skill Development
- Individual obstacle training
- Combination obstacle training

C. 5 minutes—Team Meeting
- Stress positive attitude/hard work

Part II. Preseason Training (December to March)
A. 20 minutes—Strength/Sprinter Speed/Agility Drills
- *Strength* Weight pushes with increasing weights
  10 m pullbacks
- *Speed* 50 m sprints
  Starts, finishes, body positioning
- *Agility* 30 seconds of directional changes on command

B. 20 minutes—Individual Skill Development
- Progress to combination of obstacles
  3/4/5 in a series

C. 5 minutes—Team Meeting
- Stress mental readiness and concentration

Part III. In-Season Training (April to June)
A. 10 minutes—Strength/Speed/Agility Drills
- One run per athlete in the combined four drills
- Alternate weeks—full loads and half loads

B. 30 minutes—Individual Skill Developments
- Full slalom courses: 75% of time, using standard course
  25% of time, varied obstacle course

C. 5 minutes—Team Meeting
- Review strengths and weaknesses

Practice Outside of Practice

The individual components, limited space requirements, and simply made obstacles make it very easy for athletes to practice outside of their team's organized practices. Although it will be unusual for athletes to be able to set up an entire course, they should be encouraged to practice on specific segments of the course whenever possible.

Setting Up a Program of Modified Aerobics for People With Physical Disabilities

Barbara Cancilla

Marilyn Pink

Exercise to music through jazzercise, dancercise, or aerobic workouts is becoming a popular event for men and women of all age groups. The benefits from such workouts include improved range of motion or flexibility, increased strength, increased endurance, and improved efficiency of the heart and lungs. Exercise can also improve posture, help in weight control, and lead to increased feelings of well-being. People with disabilities can benefit from this type of workout and be part of the fitness craze, too. A program of modified aerobics can be set up to meet the needs of people with disabilities.

In order to take part in an exercise program safely, the participant should be screened by a physical therapist or knowledgeable medical personnel. Information regarding the individual's past medical history and present status should be collected to modify the program to meet the individual's needs as well as to act as a baseline to monitor progress.

Screens should include a measurement of the heart's response to exercise through a stress test using an arm ergometer, a bicycle, or a treadmill. An evaluation of the individual's strength, flexibility, range of motion, chest expansion, and breathing pattern should also be done. An assessment of how the participant gets in and out of a chair, or on and off the floor, or how he or she maneuvers his or her wheelchair, will tell the "functional abilities." Individuals can be classified as *independent* (those persons who can walk and perform functional activities without assistance); *assisted* (those persons who require use of a cane, crutches, walker, or physical assistance of another person); or *wheelchair mobile* (those persons who require use of a wheelchair). A 5-minute minipracticum of exercises can also be done to see if the participant has enough endurance and coordination to take part in the group.

The physical area for a modified aerobics program should be large enough to accommodate mats, chairs, and wheelchairs with plenty of room for everyone to move around safely. The participant should wear loose-fitting cotton clothing, like a shirt and shorts, to adjust for changes in body temperature. The only equipment necessary includes a tape recorder and a watch with a second hand. The music used for these workouts should include 10 minutes of slow songs to allow for a good stretch workout and warm-up prior to the more vigorous exercises. This should be followed by a 20-minute session of fast, peppy music that will increase the heart rate. Finally, a 10-minute session of slower music should be used for cooling down and for postactivity stretching. Tapes can be made by the leaders or by the individuals. It might be more fun and stimulating to rotate the tapes each week to encourage the participants to be creative and to exercise to music they like.

Before getting into the exercise routine, the participant should be instructed in the purpose and skill of monitoring his or her heart rate. If the participant is unable to take his or her own pulse, the leader can take it at designated intervals. Based upon the individual's evaluation screen, an exercise heart rate can be taken and assigned to each participant.

Now we are ready to begin the program. The group can be divided into different classifications (i.e., those who are independent, those participants who require the assistance of a chair or wall bar to hold onto for balance, and those who are wheelchair mobile). All participants can be encouraged to join as many of the exercises as they can. Exercises can be modified to meet the needs of the participants. The leader may also want to choose one participant from each classification to act as a model for that group.

All the participants can take a resting heart rate before beginning. Ten minutes of slow stretches with the slower music should begin the program. This is done to increase the circulation and stretch out the muscles to their full range of motion in order to prevent injury to the muscles and joints during the more intense exercises. The heart rate is again taken after the stretching and warm-up to see if the participants have warmed up enough for the next section. Once warmed up, the participants are ready for 20 minutes of more intense exercises done with the fast, peppy music. These exercises include running, marching, or dancing in place; or for those in wheelchairs, the exercise includes rapid rhythmical arm exercises. Heart rates are monitored periodically throughout the more intense exercises to ensure that the participants are exercising safely. The slow music should then signal the time to cool down and to stretch again. Postactivity stretching can again help to prevent injury and muscle soreness. A final heart rate can be taken to see if each participant has returned to his or her resting level.

The above model can be modified further to meet your individual needs. It can be a great workout and lots of fun too. Enjoy!

General Ideologies and Methods of Powerlifting

Bob Accorsi
Raphael Bieber
F. John Bugbee
Fred Koch

The intention of this chapter on powerlifting is to provide coaches and athletes with an introduction to a variety of lifting programs to meet the specific needs of the individual athlete. Powerlifting programs are one of the most valuable, beneficial, and essential components for the overall development of a good athlete.

Training programs can provide the diversity that will enhance individual performance levels in any event. The following programs and methodologies are only a few of the many available, but we feel they have been proven over a period of time and are the most appropriate for the cerebral palsy (CP) athlete.

One important note to keep in mind when weight training with CP athletes is that competitive powerlifting and weight training is a bilateral event that requires balance and coordination from both sides of the body. While we encourage supervised weight training for preparation of events, we find competitive powerlifting for the hemiplegic individual dangerous and inappropriate. The unilateral use of the body by the individual causes incredible stress and strain on the joints and muscles that can cause severe damage. We recommend that any hemiplegic consult both a coach and a physical therapist before deciding if competitive lifting is appropriate.

Heavy Training and the Overload Principle

Hatfield (1981) stresses the overload principle of training as a means to increase strength and endurance in an athlete. Simply stated, the overload principle means that you force the muscle into doing something it is not accustomed to do. There are many ways to overload. Increasing the weight, reps, or sets, decreasing the rest periods, increasing the speed of movements, or increasing the speed with which the entire set is performed all will cause overloads.

Strength development is achieved by lifting weights that are as heavy as possible. The athlete and coach next need to decide what is heavy and what is light. Simply defined, heavy is the maximum amount you can lift for a required number of sets. For example, if your last rep in a set of 20 curls is an absolute maximum effort, that is heavy. Light, on the other hand, means that the weight you use allows you to perform the required number of sets without forcing you to exert maximum effort on the final rep.

The training program consists of a three-part, six-set system for each body part.

- Part 1—2 sets/6 reps/fast as possible/last rep should be maximum effort/ 1 minute rest between sets.
- Part 2—2 set/12 reps/rest between sets a few minutes/use lighter weight for these sets/use slower and controlled movements/rest again.
- Part 3—Finish off your body part routine with 2 sets—20 to 25 reps/slow continuous movements.

Remember, the keys to this program are variation and heavy poundage. Use the heaviest weight you can handle for each set, whether you do 6 or 25 reps. As your strength and endurance increases, adjust the weight accordingly.

Nautilus/Resistance Machines

The Nautilus phenomenon has swept the country in the past few years. Invented and developed by Arthur Jones in 1970, these spacelike machines are virtually in every health, racquet, and gym club in the United States. The primary purpose of Nautilus is to increase cardiovascular fitness, strength, and flexibility.

The unique feature of the Nautilus machine is that it provides full range variable resistance through very carefully designed eccentric cams or spiral pulleys. Nautilus stresses high-intensity exercise to stimulate muscle growth and increase strength. The higher the intensity, the better the stimulation. The exercise should be terminated only when additional repetitions are impossible.

Nautilus machines accentuate negative resistance as much as positive resistance. Positive work occurs during the raising of weight against gravity. Lowering the weight under control involves negative work, which is believed to be the single most important component in high-intensity exercise.

A standard program usually consists of:

- Beginners—15 to 20 minutes/entire workout; 5 machines
- Intermediate—20 to 30 minutes/entire workout; 8 machines
- Advanced—30 to 45 minutes/entire workout; 12 machines

Nautilus programs are designed to meet specific needs of every athlete. Most Nautilus instructors will assist in tailoring programs for you. Coaches should consider Nautilus or other resistance machines when designing a training program for your athlete.

Competitive Lifting

Pretraining Evaluation

A number of importance factors must be considered when deciding if an athlete will make a good competitive lifter. These include emotional desire, medical approval, cognitive understanding of training and its demands, and body structure. Body structure is one of the most important factors in predicting which athlete will be a highly competitive lifter. In bench pressing, the individual with shorter arms and barrel chests have usually outperformed those who are long-armed and flat-chested. The biomechanics of forces and leverage are in favor of the short-armed, barrel-chested lifter. Training, however, can change that.

Bench Position for Maximum Performance

Proper positioning on the bench will be a key factor to the success of your lifter. The athlete should be comfortable and balanced, which may require his or her legs to be supported. Arms should be able to hang down on the side of the bench. Benches more than 9 in. wide may prevent this from happening.

The bar or handles should be 1 in. above the nipples of the chest. Grip the bar slightly more than shoulder width. As a lifter trains, he or she will find his or her maximum width and still perform well. Coaches should measure exact width for future information. Watch that the heel of the hand and wrist are at a right angle to the bar. Fingers should be tight, and the wrist straight and locked. You want the weight to pass down through the forearms, not the fingers or hand.

The lifter's head should be in a natural resting position, not twisted or leaning to any one side. Body alignment is extremely important. The head should not rise off the bench during lifts because it is illegal in competition. The use of Universals may require that you adjust the athlete so his or her head clears the travel of the weights.

Training Hints

Whenever possible, it is suggested that you train with a partner. This will provide some additional motivation as well as help make workouts more enjoyable. Be careful not to overtrain. Give yourself a minimum of 3 days of rest per week and stay away from doing single reps too often. Also, do not restrict your lifting to just bench press. Developing a sound base of strength in all the muscles surrounding the shoulder area will help you not only develop a great bench press, but also keep you competitive for many years to come.

Also, do not forget the importance of supplementing your lifting program with a well-rounded flexibility and stretching program. Powerlifting represents a very explosive activity for which you must properly prepare the muscles.

A good flexibility routine should be done prior to and immediately after a workout, as well as be a part of your preparation for competition. Refer to the section on flexibility for more specifics.

Breathing

A lifter's breathing pattern represents one of the most important final preparations a lifter can make before actually making the lift. As in any other sport, a lifter's final preparation should become a consistent routine. Once in position on the bench with good head alignment and proper hand positioning on the bar, the lifter should take three deep breaths while relaxing the body and making a mental image of exactly how the lift should and will be done. On the fourth breath, the lifter should inhale deeply and begin the lift as he or she slowly exhales. The lift and the exhaling should be simultaneous. The lifter should not expel all the air and should attempt to maintain an expanded rib cage.

The Role of Repetitions

Many lifters may be accustomed to training with a greater number of repetitions than indicated within this article. These suggestions for repetitions are based on the following assumptions:

1. 15 or more reps: usually done to promote cardiovascular fitness and muscle endurance.
2. 8 to 15 reps: usually done by body builders seeking to pump up their muscles. Up to a certain point, the more reps you perform, the faster fatigue products will build up and the greater the blood flow to your muscles will be. Although this method has a very stimulating effect on muscles, it does not allow you to handle heavy weight, thus reducing the potential for strength increases. High repetitions may also increase spasticity in some CP athletes.
3. 3 to 7 reps: working within this range of repetitions allows you to handle heavy weight and stimulate a maximum number of muscle fibers. The reps are low enough that any excessive pumping is avoided. Thus the emphasis is on the development of strength, not building inflated tissues.
4. 1 to 2 reps: used for testing strength rather than building strength.

6-Month Training Program

The following is an *example* program for preparing a beginning lifter for a competition that is 6 months away. This routine may *not* work for everyone; in fact, individualized programs are a must in order to get the best from each lifter. Do not attempt to have everyone on one schedule or routine. A more experienced lifter should be on a more aggressive program.

- Month 6   5 sets—max—8 reps
- Month 5   1st set—warm-up—8 reps
    2nd set—5 reps
    3rd set—5 reps
    4th set—5 reps
    5th set—3 reps
    6th set—every 2 to 3 weeks max top end lifting
- Month 4   1st set—warm-up—8 reps
    2nd set—5 reps
    3rd set—5 reps
    4th set—3 to 5 reps—forced
- Month 3   1st set—warm-ups—8 reps
    2nd set—5 reps
    3rd set—3 to 5 reps—forced
    4th set—3 to 5 reps—forced
    5th set—1 to 3 reps—forced
- Month 2   1st set—warm-ups—8 reps
    2nd set—5 reps
    3rd set—1 to 3 reps—forced reps 2 to 3
    5th set—5 reps—less weight so lifter can lift independently

Forced reps are repetitions where the lifter can only do two or three on his own and with assistance completes the five. The assistance is very little, and the lifter is "tortured" into successful repetitions. *Never* hurt your lifter by not assisting enough; making him or her fight to push the weight makes his or her muscles "burn," but do not overstrain your lifter.

Four weeks from competition, suggest your lifter perform this program (top end as in a contest):

- 1st set—8 reps—warm-ups
- 2nd set—1 rep—weight lifter can easily and usually make 80% of top end
- 3rd set—1 rep—90% of top end weight
- 4th set—100% of top end
- 5th set—5 to 10 lb over top end

You should intend to win a competition with your second lift. The third lift should be the amount or personal best for that individual. This amount may have only been successfully made once or twice before. Another approach is based on percentages; for example, the first lift can be made 100% of the times attempted, the second lift 80 to 90% of the times attempted, and the third lift 25 to 50% of the times.

The final weeks of training must be based on individual needs. Some lifters need only 1 week of rest while others require 2 or more.

Three weeks from competition, a lifter can perform the following:

- 1st set—8 reps—warm-up
- 2nd, 3rd, 4th sets—1 rep—forced total breaking down of lifter's strength, barely makes 85% of top end

Two weeks from competition should be a time of rest, with no lifting. One week from competition, the lifter may do light workouts of 5 sets, 3 to 5 reps at 40, 60, and 80% of top end. The workout should be very easy for the lifter. The lifter should feel as if the weight is *too light*. If strain occurs, give more time off or reduce weight and reps.

During the week of competition, if the contest takes place on Saturday, the lifter should have a light workout on Monday (5 sets at 40, 60, 80, and 90%). On Wednesday, consider the workout a dress rehearsal for Saturday's competition. The first set should be warming up. The second set should consist of a first competitive lift, 1 rep; a second competitive lift, 1 rep; and a third competitive lift, top end. Duplicate all rules and pressure of competition (which you should have been doing all along). If your lifter makes all three lifts you can be sure he or she is prepared physically for competition. If he or she missed the second lift, evaluate all competitive weights to be attempted. If your lifter just misses the third lift, stick with it. He or she may get psyched up during competiton and make it.

Remember, the routine given may work for several lifters—*but not for all*. Research and educate yourself and prepare.

Note

For additional information contact: Powerlifting U.S.A., Box 467, Camarillo, CA 93011 or National Strength & Conditioning Association, P.O. Box 81410, Lincoln, NE 68501, (402) 472-3000.

Additional Readings

Accorsi, B., Bugbee, R.J., Koch, F. (1984). *General ideologies and methods of powerlifting, Training guide to cerebral palsy sports*, (2nd ed.). NY: United Cerebral Palsy Association, Inc.

Hatfield, F.C. (1981). *Powerlifting: A scientific approach.* Chicago: Contemporary Books.

Koch, F. (1980). *Weightlifting techniques. A training guide to all aspects of cerebral palsy sports.* NY: United Cerebral Palsy Association, Inc.

McLaughlin, T.M. (1984). *Bench press more now: Breakthrough in biomechanics and training methods.* Roswell, GA: Author.

Weight Training: The Key to Individual Event Success

Scott Cusimano
Ron Davis

Weight training has become a very popular method of preparing for athletic competition. Much has been accomplished by using weight training to contribute to improved physical performance within a sporting event. Gone are the myths of becoming a muscle-bound hulk incapable of performing something as graceful as a floor exercise routine in gymnastics or a flip turn in swimming. It is not generally accepted that under proper supervision, gymnasts, swimmers, basketball players, and others are significantly improving their athletic performances through the use of weight training.

Disabled athletes should also be given every opportunity to improve their athletic endeavors. If coaches for disabled athletes are concerned about the development of their athletes, the use of weight training appears inevitable.

The remainder of this chapter deals with specific weight training exercises for events of cerebral palsy (CP) sports. The objective of this chapter is to provide the athlete and the coach a guide for implementing weight training exercises designed to develop those muscle groups specific to the skill. Careful consideration has been taken in the selection of the exercises for each event; however, the user is free to rearrange the exercises according to individual team needs and desires.

Training Concepts

The coach must decide which approaches to weight training are appropriately suited for his or her individual athletes or team. Weight training programs can be emphasized to improve power, muscular endurance, and/or maintain strength. A sample program is provided later to give the user guidelines for a power or muscular endurance or a strength maintenance emphasis.

Overload Principle

The term *weight training* refers to a desire to improve physical fitness or muscular strength for a particular sporting event. Muscular strength and muscular endurance must be improved through the application of the overload principle. There must be an external resistance created in order for the muscle or muscle groups involved to work beyond normal requirements for movement. Few modern sports overload the muscles with a heavy resistance: consequently, few sports build strength.

Power

Power can be developed by using 50% of the athlete's maximum lifting strength 10 times and concentrating on good form and speed throughout the repetitions. Strength can also be developed along these guidelines with less emphasis on the speed component. For the second set, weight is added and the number of repetitions is decreased to eight. For the third set, more weight is added and the number of repetitions is decreased to six. If a fourth set is desired, the repetitions would be decreased to four with an additional weight increase.

Muscular Endurance

Low resistance and a high number of repetitions develops muscular endurance. The athlete should be able to start with a weight he or she can manage for a minimum of 10 to 12 repetitions. Some weight trainers advocate no increase in weight with each set; others indicate a small increase in weight for each set.

Strength Development/Maintenance

A well-rounded weight training program serves to develop and maintain strength. A maintenance program should include stretching exercises and nonequipment type exercises such as sit-ups and pull-ups to complement the weight training program.

Safety Guidelines

In order for any weight training program to be successful, proper safety procedures must exist. Safety is especially important when weight training with the CP athlete. The following guidelines should be enforced:

1. Never allow an athlete to lift alone or unsupervised. Always provide a spotter when free weights are being used.
2. Keep general workout area clean and free of obstacles that might cause stumbling or falling.
3. Make sure each athlete lifts under control with slow, smooth, continuous movement and insist on proper breathing during exercise. The athlete should concentrate on movement through as much range of motion as possible.
3. Avoid sudden stretching with spastic athletes that might trigger a strong muscle contraction (stretch reflex).
5. Avoid fatiguing the CP athlete with too many exercises, too much resistance, or too many repetitions.
6. Become familiar with as much of the athlete's medical background as possible.
7. Seek the advice of an adapted physical educator or physical therapist regarding correct positioning of the athlete during specific lifts.

Manual Directions

One core program has been designed with approximately 30 exercises included. They are described here as Figures 1 through 29. Most of the exercises require specific weight training equipment, whereas several need no equipment at all. Athletes should consult a doctor or physical therapist before performing these weight training exercises.

A written explanation for each exercise is provided to give the user a general idea of how the exercise should be performed. Each chart includes the categories: no equipment, free weight, Nautilus, and Universal. The user will find the name of the exercise and then an X to indicate the equipment suggested for implementation of that exercise. These are merely suggestions. The user is allowed to make changes whenever it is deemed appropriate. In addition, the same philosophy is true regarding program emphasis. The user may want to initiate a power program rather than an endurance program, and he or she has the freedom to do so. The sample program provided in Table 1 is merely to be used as a guideline. Sample swimming programs for other sports appear in Table 2.

Table 1   Sample Program for Front Crawl Swimming, Performing Lateral Pulls and Bent-Over Flies

Program emphasis	Sets	Reps	Resistance
Power	3	10, 8, 6	Increase weight each set (5 to 10 lb.)
Endurance	3	10, 12, 15	No increase of weight
Maintain strength	3	10, 10, 10	Slight increase of weight each set

Table 2   Event and Program Charts

Event	Exercise	No equipment	Free weights	Nautilus	Universal
Archery	Lateral dumbbell raises		X		
	Alternate front raises		X		
	Bent-over flies		X		
	Lateral pulls				X
	Wide grip pull-ups	X			
Swimming					
Front crawl	Lateral pulls				X
	Bent-over flies		X		
Backstroke	Leg extension			X	X
	Leg curl			X	X
	Pull-overs		X		
	Bent-over rows		X		
Breaststroke	Flat bench		X		
	Vertical leg press			X	X
	Incline sit-ups	X			
Bowling	Lateral dumbbell raises		X		
	Alternate front raises		X		
	Bent-over flies		X		
	Shrugs		X		X
Horseback riding					
Posting	Vertical leg press			X	X
	Half squats		X		
	Side bends	X	X		
Wheelchair events					
Slalom	Triceps extension		X	X	
	Shrugs		X		
	Lateral dumbbell		X		
	Alternate front raises		X		
	Bent-over flies		X		
Racing-arms (same as slalom in addition)					
	Flat bench		X		X
	Incline bench		X	X	
	Dips	X			X
	Decline sit-ups	X			X
	Incline crunches	X			X
Long jump	Half squats		X		
	Leg extension			X	X
	Leg curl			X	X

(Cont.)

Table 2 (Cont.)

Event	Exercise	No equipment	Free weights	Nautilus	Universal
Weight lifting					
Bench press	Flat bench		X	X	X
	Incline bench		X		
	Military press		X	X	X
	Tricep extension		X		
	Push-downs				X
Ambulatory racing					
Crutches	Flat bench		X	X	X
	Lateral dumbbell raises		X		
	Alternate front raises		X		
	Bent-over flies		X		
	Shrugs		X		X
	Dips		X		
Nonassisted racing					
	Half squats		X		
	Leg extension			X	X
	Leg curl			X	X
	Flat bench		X	X	X
	Lateral dumbbell raises		X		
	Alternate front raises		X		
	Bent-over flies		X		
	Pull-overs (DB)		X		
	Incline sit-ups	X			X
	Decline leg raises	X			X
Cycling and tricycling					
	Half squats		X		
	Vertical leg press				X
	Leg extension			X	X
	Leg curl			X	X
	Lateral pulls				X
	Wide grip pull-ups	X			X
	Concentrated dumbbell curls		X		
	Incline sit-ups	X			X
	Side bends	X	X		
	Flat bench		X	X	X
	Push-downs				X

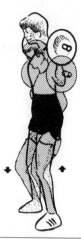

Figure 1. Half squats. Bar either in a squat rack or free, bar across back of shoulders, squat to 70 to 90° flexion at knees.

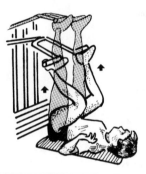

Figure 2. Vertical leg press. Using bench press station on Universal machine or the equivalent, lie flat on back with feet underneath handles, press legs to full extension, then return, repeat.

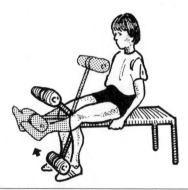

Figure 3. Leg extension. Position feet in padded rollers. Alternate leg extensions at knee for full extension. Hold each extension for 2 seconds.

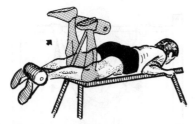

Figure 4.   Leg curl. Same machine as in Figure 3; lie on stomach, hook ankles on upper padded rollers, alternate pulling heels to buttocks, hold for 2 seconds then return, repeat.

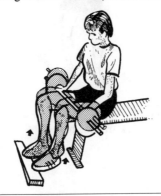

Figure 5.   Toe raises. Position weight across shoulders, or remain seated with weight across knees. Position feet on an uneven surface with balls of feet slightly higher than heels (approximately 1 to 2 in.). Using only the toes, lift heels up, then return. Repeat exercise with feet in three positions, toes facing out, toes facing inward, toes straight ahead.

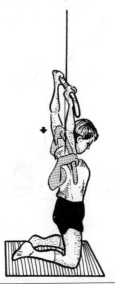

Figure 6.   Lateral pulls. Using long cross bar on a cable (Universal machine), sit or kneel with wide grip, pull bar behind head, then slowly return to start.

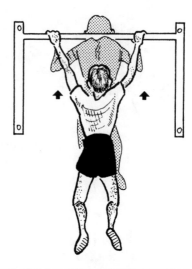

Figure 7. Wide grip pull-ups. Hanging from cross bar with palms away from body, pull body up, touch bar to back of neck, return, repeat.

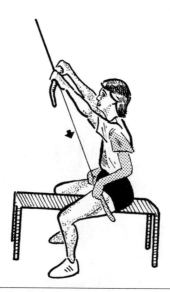

Figure 8. Incline waist pulls. Sitting on an incline bench, facing Universal machine, same station at lateral pulls, pull bar down to waist.

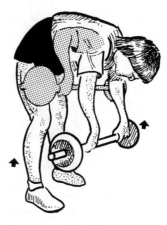

Figure 9. Bent-over rows. Place free weight barbell on floor, bend forward to pull bar to chest, return slowly to floor, repeat.

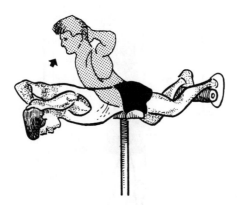

Figure 10. Prone arches. Using prone arch station of Universal machine or similar hip support and feet rest, lay over pad and then arch entire body past horizontal, return.

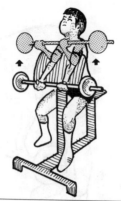

Figure 11.   Chest curls. Using a curl bar or regular barbell, use heavier weight than normal, palms up, curl bar to chest. Extra body movement is allowed to accomplish heavy weight.

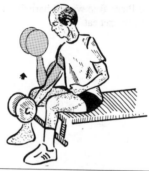

Figure 12.   Concentrated dumbbell curls. Use dumbbells either on "preacher seat" or individually in each hand, curl weight with elbows supported on bench.

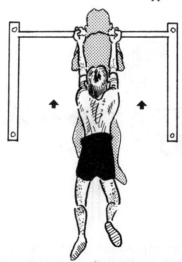

Figure 13.   Close grip chin-up. On same bar as pull-ups, hands one width apart, palms to body, pull up, touch chin to bar, repeat.

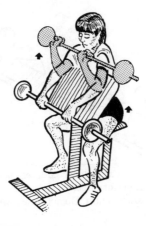

Figure 14. Reverse curls. Same as chest curls but hands are turned over (palms away).

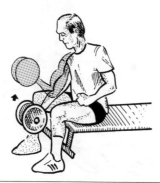

Figure 15. Biceps "21s." Sitting on the end of a bench, with a dumbbell in each hand, leave elbows stationary, curl weight up to 90° at elbow, then down, do 7 reps, then start weight vertical at shoulder, lower from shoulder to 90° at elbow, do 7 reps, then full range of motion, do 7 reps (7 + 7 + 7 = 21).

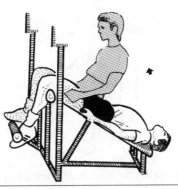

Figure 16. Roman chair sit-ups. Using a roman chair or the equivalent, lower about 20° lower than horizontal, then sit up.

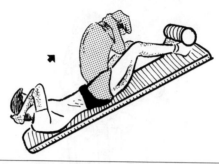

Figure 17. Decline sit-ups. Using an incline board, legs bent, do full range-of-motion sit-ups. Also on an incline board, perform incline crunches. Legs are bent slowly, roll just head and shoulders up, then slowly return. Do not raise lower back or midback off board.

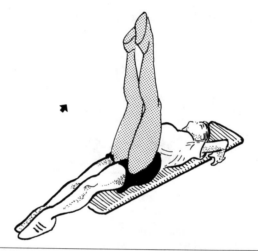

Figure 18. Decline leg raises. Using incline board, head at top, flex at waist to raise legs to the head.

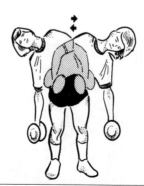

Figure 19. Side bends. Dumbbell in one hand, bend sideways until weight is below knees, then alternate left to right.

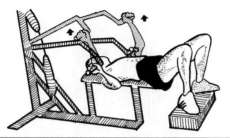

Figure 20.   Flat bench. Using flat bench, either free weight or Universal machine, bench press full range of motion with hands on fist wider than shoulder width.

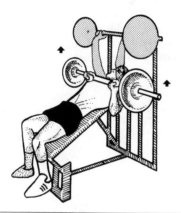

Figure 21.   Incline bench. Same principles as flat bench except use an incline bench instead of a flat bench. Start with a lighter weight.

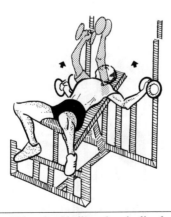

Figure 22.   Incline flies. Using dumbbells and an incline bench, start with weight over chest, palms facing inward, slowly let weight down, outward until weight is even or lower than chest. Return to starting position, repeat.

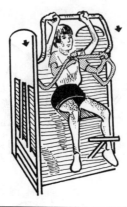

Figure 23.   Pull-overs. Start with dumbbell on floor, lie with shoulders (perpendicular) on flat bench (supine). Reach behind head and pull weight with both hands over head to chest, arms slightly bent, then return and repeat.

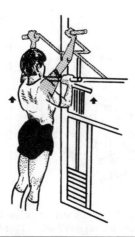

Figure 24.   Military press. Using Universal machine or free weight, sit, then press from chest to over head. Do 2 sets facing weight, 2 sets facing away.

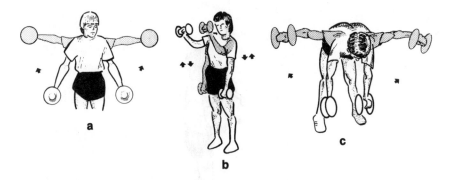

Figure 25. Dumbbell raises (a). Standing with dumbbell in each hand, weight at side, raise weight (straight arms) up to horizontal. Weights must stay to the side, not to the front. Alternate front raises (b). Same starting position as above, move weight to position in front (on thighs). Raise one hand (straight arms) to horizontal, alternate left, right. Repeat. Bent-over flies (c). Bend forward at waist, back flat, with dumbbells in each hand, raise weight up and outward (similar to incline flies) with arm slightly bent. Repeat.

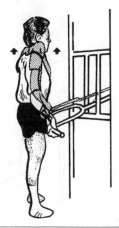

Figure 26. Shrugs. Using heavy weight, either free or Universal machine, keep arms straight, weight in hands, lift with shoulders, shrug up, then down. Repeat.

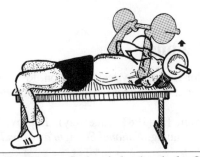

Figure 27. Triceps extension. Using a flat bench, hands only 6 to 8 in. apart with weight held in a bench press position bending only at the elbows, lower weight to forehead, then return to start. Do 2 sets with palms facing body, 2 sets with palms facing away.

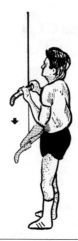

Figure 28. Push-downs. Using lat machine (Universal) hands together, palms down, push bar down until arms are fully extended, then slowly return to start.

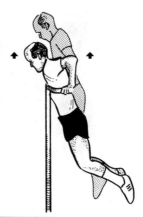

Figure 29. Dips. Using dip station on Universal machine or even parallel bars, bend elbows to lower body to bar height, then extend arms to starting position. The feet should not touch the floor.

Additional Readings

American Alliance for Health, Physical Education, Recreation and Dance. (1978, December). Weight training for wheelchair sports. *Practical Pointers, 2*(6), 7–16.

Burke, E., & Newton, H. (1983, June/July). Improved cycling performance through strength training. *National Strength and Conditioning Journal, 5* (3), 6–7, 70–71.

Hooks, G. (1974). *Weight training in athletics and physical education.* Englewood Cliffs, NJ: Prentice-Hall.

Training Riders for Competition

Natalie Bieber

Anyone interested in learning to ride a horse for pleasure, therapy, or sport should understand that good riding is the result of mutual confidence and effort on the parts of the rider, the horse and the instructor/coach. It is also a result of being taught the correct thing to do and doing it over and over again until muscles accommodate and strengthen and reactions become automatic. Learning time is a variable that all riders face, whether disabled or not, and is strongly influenced by both motivation and saddle time. The prime aim of good riding instruction is a secure seat on the horse. Once this is achieved, the student can move ahead to advanced aspects of performance and competition. Riding can be the basis for a whole rehabilitation program, but this discussion will focus on those points that are relevant to horseback riding as a sport. It is enough to comment that it is a perceptibly healthy exercise that stimulates respiration, circulation, and muscular activity and enhances coordination, balance, and endurance.

Horseback riding may not be an appropriate choice for every person. A physician's approval should be obtained prior to engaging in any riding activity. However, no special physical attributes are necessary. You don't have to be young, thin, tall, or short, just willing and patient. The rider should have realistic goals and realize that progress is not measured only in terms of gait and speed of the horse, but also in the amount of independent action on the part of the rider and the complexity of movements that can be performed. Riding is as appropriate a sport for a Class I cerebral palsy (CP) athlete as for a Class VIII. The demands of the events will differ, but the challenge remains. The equestrian events included in United States Cerebral Palsy Athletic Association (USCPAA) competitions are dressage, equitation, obstacle course, relay race, and jumping. Novice and advanced sections for riders of different classifications are encouraged at the local and regional levels to enable as many persons as possible to get all-important ring experience.

Special Concerns

Riding should be undertaken under the guidance of a coach or instructor who is thoroughly horse knowledgeable and can properly match the rider, horse, and tack (equipment). This person should have an awareness of the special needs of physically disabled individuals and have support in the form of a physical therapist and volunteers to be leaders and sidewalkers as needed. The ideal instructor is one who has experience coaching nondisabled riders for competition as well as working with riders with disabilities. A riding lesson for a CP rider should have the same basic components as one for any nondisabled rider. The instructor must, however, exercise special vigilance with regard to safety and fatigue factors without adding the overprotective element that might stifle challenge and development. Because all riding involves the element of controlled risk, it is extremely important that the instructor waits to proceed with the introduction of any new skill, whether it is going from the walk to the trot or removing a sidewalker or leader, until he or she is sure that the prerequisite skills have been mastered. Effective riding lessons do not just happen; they are the result of thought and organization on the part of the instructor. Ideally, the time frame for a riding session should be 1 1/2 hours if a rider with a physical disability is to receive maximum benefits. The mounted portion of the time should include passive and active exercise, instruction in technique, and purely recreational components.

Preparation

Mounting the rider should be undertaken with the unique needs of the individual in mind. It may necessitate the use of a ramp, mounting block, and/or several helpers (see Figure 1). Positioning during mounting should inhibit any tendency toward hyperextension and facilitate appropriate flexion. Once the rider is mounted, no quick attempt should be made to place the feet in the stirrups or

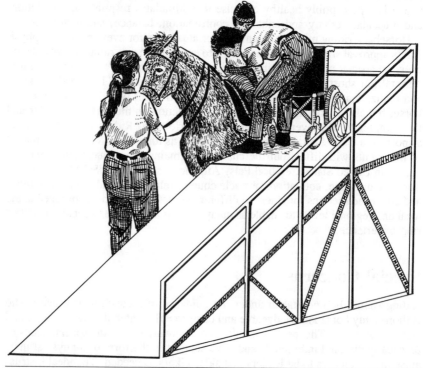

Figure 1. Using a ramp for mounting a wheelchair participant.

to position the legs. Where there is spasticity with internal rotation, extensor thrust, or severe scissoring, the rider should be given ample time to be relaxed by the motion of the horse before anything else is attempted.

The time allotment for the warm-up phase of an ideal riding session is influenced by many variables. Each rider is different and each lesson will be different. Riding should always be viewed as a dynamic interaction, and weather and mood can affect relaxation time as much as physical attributes. The rider may initially need external stabilization in the form of sidewalkers' support or self-support holding onto a strap attached to the saddle. Perhaps 10 minutes at the walk should be sufficient before proceeding to the more demanding phases of the ride.

The second mounted activity pertains to the development of skills and endurance. During this phase of the lesson, riding techniques are presented and practiced. The rider now actively assumes the responsibility for the horse's performance and is encouraged to use arms, legs, and seat to control the direction and forward motion of the mount. Work at the walk, trot, halt, circles, and change of direction should be included. It is appropriate to give special attention to use of aids and transitions from one gait to another. The most important objective for the riding instructor is to get the rider to focus on the immediate goal and not think of other things.

When working on positioning the hands, forget about the heels. Most importantly, the rider must keep the eyes up, looking at some point ahead. Looking down throws the entire body out of balance. The rider must try to think about what the horse is doing. The horse moves up and down, laterally, and diagonally under the rider. The principal aims are to coordinate successive movements, to train reaction capability, and to develop a deep seat.

When the rider reaches the point where he or she has sufficient stability in the saddle and does not use the reins for balance and support, he or she can learn to use the rein as an aid. The reins should be held in the closest approximation of standard position as possible. Through the reins, and therefore the hands, the rider regulates pace and directs the horse. Most of the horse's training depends on its mouth, and the rider must learn to give and take with his or her hands. Educated hands use a squeezing motion that becomes a reflex action. Specially adapted reins are available for persons who cannot grasp standard ones—ladder and Humes are two—and these should be used when needed (see Figure 2).

The next step in developing riding skills involves making the horse move forward according to the rider's wishes. The legs should not be used to kick the horse, only squeeze; kicking disturbs the rider's balance and lessens his or her safety. Where functional ability precludes using the legs, the rider should try pushing down with the seat to urge the horse on and/or use a crop. In learning to use the elementary aids, it is important to spend a lot of time at the walk while the rider feels the kinds of effects the different aids produce. Unfortunately, many instructors of disabled riders do not emphasize this enough. Riders should not be allowed to develop sloppy techniques because of their disabilities.

Mounted Activities

Once stability and balance have been established at the walk, the rider can progress to the sitting trot. An understanding of the cause and effect that underlies all good

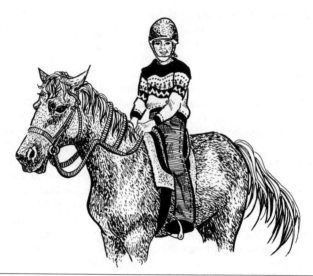

Figure 2.   Ladder reins are used with riders that have difficulties grasping standard reins.

equitation needs to be emphasized at the cognitive as well as the physical level. It may be necessary to master the skills learned at the walk all over again at the trot due to the difference in rhythm and speed between the two gaits. The need for practice and patience at this point cannot be overemphasized. The posting trot, moving out of the saddle in cadence with the diagonal movement of the horse's legs, is a skill that some disabled riders may never achieve (Figure 3). For those unable to accomplish this, it should be noted that they will not be marked down in horsemanship. Being able to sit quietly and well at the sitting trot gives the most elegant impression and is a skill scored high in competition.

It is advisable to spend specific time on the movements included in dressage. It is during this phase of a riding session that most of the prerequisite skills for competition should be taught and practiced. The object of dressage is the harmonious development of the horse and the achievement of perfect understanding with its rider. The rider should direct the horse so that it gives the impression of doing the pattern of movements in the dressage test of its own accord. Practice is required to achieve a precise and fluent dressage ride. This is excellent training for both horse and rider as they learn to work together as a team. The following are tips for training riders for dressage competition:

- Teach and practice individual movements before trying to ride the entire test.
- Because of possible perceptual problems, it is important to diagram the figures on paper, and then work on them mounted, giving both visual and kinesthetic feedback.
- The rider should practice the pattern unmounted in order to memorize it.
- The whole test should not be overdrilled when mounted because this can result in a loss of spontaneity on the part of the horse.

Always remember that dressage is scored on a combination of performance by horse and rider, though emphasis is placed on the rider in CP sports.

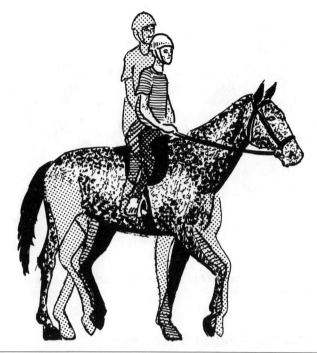

Figure 3.   Posting while walking or trotting is a skill some riders will not be able to achieve.

The skill/endurance phase of the lesson should take from 15 to 30 minutes. Again, the time will be influenced by the variables mentioned before, as well as the number of riders in the group, their stamina, and the need for individualized attention. A class with more than six disabled riders with their assorted leaders and sidewalkers in the ring at once can reduce a well-planned lesson to a "pony ride."

The third mounted activity involves exercises. These should be prescribed by a physical therapist, but could include the "monkey" drills commonly used by instructors for nondisabled populations to develop balance, flexibility, and the deep, secure seat so essential if a rider is to be more than a passenger. Balance exercises should start with the horse stationary and progress to those at the walk when appropriate. Figure 4 depicts some exercises that are used fairly routinely with CP and other riders. One cautionary note however: Not all exercises are appropriate for all riders. The advice of a physical therapist is important to ensure that exercises do not trigger the abnormal reflex patterns that the riding session can suppress, especially where the CP rider is concerned.

The final 10 to 15 minutes of the session should be recreational. The rider has had warm-up time, skill development, and structured exercise. For riders with the desire to compete in horse shows or USCPAA competition, relay races and obstacle courses are appropriate for this portion of the class. Fast and slow walking races are fun for riders at both the novice and advanced levels. It is often easier to teach important elements of technique and achieve success in a recreational context. The riders are relaxed and often wind up doing subconsciously the very thing that was worked on at the conscious level. The final phase of the

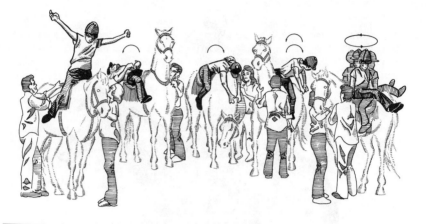

Figure 4. Common exercises used with CP riders.

ride should be structured for fun and to afford each rider an opportunity to experience personal success.

Developing a Winning Attitude

Both the rider and instructor should have realistic goals that provide the opportunities for challenge and success. Many equestrian events are at the walk and trot. Competence is not necessarily measured in terms of gait or speed of the horse. The two most important things for the physically disabled rider to strive for are independence and precision. The severely involved rider who can do a precise dressage test at the walk is as skilled as the less disabled person who does this at the trot or canter.

To compete successfully, riders must not only master the techniques and rules for their events, but also be "ring wise." Some equestrian events are judged rather subjectively, so it is important for the competitor to realize that the overall impression he or she makes on the judge can be as important as the performance. Neatness of attire is a must. The rider should be relaxed, but businesslike, and project a picture of competency and enjoyment. In a class with a group of riders, he or she should avoid being blocked from the judge's view by another horse and rider. He or she should be alert for the instructions of the ringmaster. Transitions from one gait to another should be prompt but not hurried or sloppy. Minor performance mistakes should be subtly corrected. The more polished the performance, the better the chance of winning.

Most riders find that they are capable of doing much more than they ever dreamed was possible. With good instruction, patience, and ample time in the saddle, progress will continue. Competition adds spice to the joys of riding. Winning requires practice, perseverance, precision, and patience. No matter what the event, enter the ring like a winner in order to be one!

Note

The purpose of this training guide is primarily to provide a general overview of the sports available to athletes with CP. Equestrian competition represents the most complicated and difficult sport to coach within the USCPAA umbrella. It is the opinion of this editor that whenever possible, local programs should solicit the expertise of national governing bodies and/or local college or high school coaches. In respect to horseback riding, there are two excellent sources of expertise: The American Horse Shows Association, Inc., 598 Madison Ave., New York, NY 10022, (212) 759-3070 and North American Riding for the Handicapped Association, Inc., 111 E. Walker Drive, Suite 600, Chicago, IL 60601, (312) 644-6610. NARHA represents more than 150 accredited therapeutic riding programs nationwide and can provide anyone thinking of beginning a riding program or wanting to know about local accredited programs a great deal of guidance and reference materials.

Additional Reading

McCowan, L.L. (1972). *It is ability that counts: A training manual on therapeutic riding for the handicapped.* Olivet, MI: Olivet College Press.

Archery

MaryBeth Jones

It is difficult to estimate the numbers of individuals with cerebral palsy (CP) that actively participate in archery. Although the numbers of competitors in archery events at national competitions have been quite small, a great many more seem to be enjoying archery in recreation programs across the country. The purpose of this chapter is to provide coaches and athletes with some general information on equipment, training, shooting techniques, and safety while also providing a number of excellent references for additional information. It should be understood from the beginning that, whether you choose to participate in archery recreationally or competitively, the practices and policies of able-bodied archery will be the foundation from which to begin. However, they by no means represent the only way to enjoy the sport of archery.

It is important to seek the assistance of an experienced archer or coach when first beginning in archery. Contacting local archery clubs or shops would be the first place to begin. If those resources are not available within your immediate area, contact the National Archery Association for information about local programs within your community.

Equipment

The general rule of thumb suggests that you try archery several times before you consider buying your own equipment. If you then decide to pursue archery as a sport, you should purchase your own equipment in order to meet your individual needs (see Figure 1).

Bows

If you consult with an experienced archer, you should be advised to be prudent when selecting your first bow (Figure 2). The primary difference between one

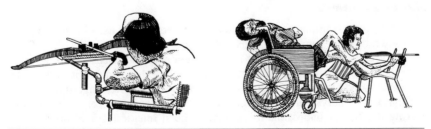

Figure 1. Different abilities within different individuals will require coaches to be creative when developing adapted equipment.

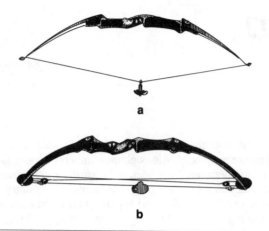

Figure 2. Types of bows. A conventional recurve bow with shooting release (a), and compound bow with finger tab (b).

bow and another is what is called poundage, pull, or a bow's weight. This is directly related to the amount of effort that is required to draw the bow string. A bow with a 25-lb pull is much easier to use than a bow with a 40-lb pull. Beginning with a lighter pull will enhance learning because you will not be expending enormous amounts of energy or concentration trying to pull the bow string. Instead, emphasis can be put toward developing proper and consistent technique.

Once competence has been acquired with a lighter bow, you may wish to graduate up to a heavier bow that will deliver an arrow much more accurately and farther, two necessary factors if you are interested in United States Cerebral Palsy Athletic Association (USCPAA) competition. Most good archery shops have a trade-in policy, which may reduce the cost of your first and/or second bow.

Compound bows may also be useful in your transition to a heavier bow. Although the use of a compound bow is restricted in competition to only athletes in Class I and II and athletes who are severely quadraplegic (some Class VI athletes), it remains a valuable training tool. Besides being able to adjust the weight or poundage of a compound bow, once at full draw the archer is only holding half the bow's weight or poundage. Both factors allow you to gradually increase a bow's weight concurrently with the increase in your own skill and strength.

Shooting Releases

One of the most common and effective pieces of equipment used in archery, but often absent from CP archery classes is the finger tabs or shooting releases. Both devices greatly increase the ability to effectively hold and release the bowstring from the fingertips. Lack of fine motor skills of the hand makes it impossible for some individuals with CP to use the conventional three fingertip drawing method. Often individuals end up grasping the bowstring as seen in Figure 3a, making it virtually impossible to facilitate a good release (Figure 3b).

A good release is achieved by relaxing the fingers. A finger tab will provide a smoother and more uniform surface on which the bowstring can slide. Shooting

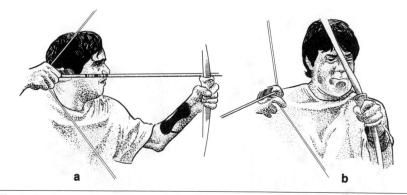

a   b

Figure 3. Fine motor problems often make a three-fingertip draw and smooth release impossible for individuals with CP.

releases provide the easiest and most effective method of drawing and releasing the bowstring. Both the finger tabs and shooting releases are shown in Figure 2. It should be noted that although shooting releases are only allowed to be used by Class I and II athletes for competition, they can be an important piece of equipment for any archer interested in recreational shooting.

Additional archery equipment such as arrows, finger tabs, bow stabilizers, bow sights, "kiss button," and hand slings will also be available at most archery shops.

Adaptive Equipment

Archery for the individuals with CP is primarily based on able-bodied technique; however, adaptations may be necessary to assist the individual to successfully participate in the sport. The suggestions and adaptations explained within this chapter are by no means the only ones available. It should be noted that certain adapted equipment is not allowed in competition; but is presented here because of the large number of individuals interested in archery solely as a recreational sport. Those archers interested in competitive shooting should consult current USCPAA archery rules to determine if their equipment is appropriate for sanctioned competition.

In developing assistive devices for your athlete, coaches must keep in mind that the adaptive equipment should be designed to *assist* the athlete in shooting and *not to replace the skill of archery with mechanical devices*. As shown in Figure 4a, the adapted equipment is only used to support the bow; the task of aiming, drawing the string, and releasing still belongs to the archer. The assistive device in Figure 4b is, in fact, an unconventional method of holding the bow. Assisted by his or her coach, the archer secures the placement of the bow on his or her feet. All lateral and horizontal movements of the bow, length of draw, and wheelchair positioning are completely within the control of the archer.

Adapted equipment can also be very specific in respect to a given problem or disability. For instance, a great deal of work has been done in the last few years by the staff of The Courage Center in Golden Valley, Minnesota in the area of upper extremity supports for individuals with severe paralysis and/or spasticity.

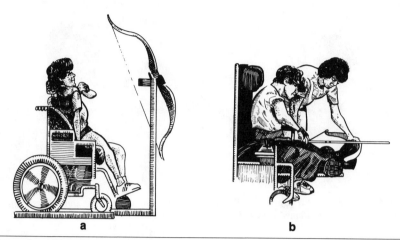

Figure 4. Although the adapted equipment is used to support the bow, the skill of archery is left up to participant (a). The same is true in (b); the coach helps to support the bow while the archer aims and shoots.

Their work includes development of adapted devices called "release cuffs" (see Figure 5a) and "bow cuffs" (see Figure 5b); both are designed specifically for individuals that do not possess the finger and wrist function necessary to either draw the bowstring or hold a bow. As a supplement to the wrist supports, they have also developed a number of elbow supports, as seen in Figure 6. Elbow supports vary from forearm to full-arm braces, depending on the archer's arm function and wrist strength.

Although use of wrist cuffs and elbow supports were initially developed for spinal cord injured quadraplegics, the potential for cross-disability use is obvious. The hemiplegic CP with a weak wrist on the "bow arm" or the athetoid CP who has difficulty maintaining fine motor control during the draw phase may want to consider the use of some type of wrist and arm supports.

Body Positioning

Regardless if the archer is ambulatory or in a wheelchair, the basic body positioning will be the same for most CP athletes involved. Those who are ambulatory will, of course, stand with their feet shoulder width apart and their bow arms and shoulders aligned directly into the center of the target. Ambulatory participants with balance difficulties should consider sitting in a chair while shooting.

Positioning a wheelchair archer for shooting is as easy as aiming the axles of the rear wheels with the center of the target, as seen in Figure 7. Although this positioning will be appropriate for most archers, the shooting styles and adapted equipment used by some CP archers (Figures 1 and 4) may require alignment of the archer's wheelchair at a variety of angles as well as straight on. Whatever position you choose, always know where your wheelchair is aimed so that portion of your technique will remain consistent.

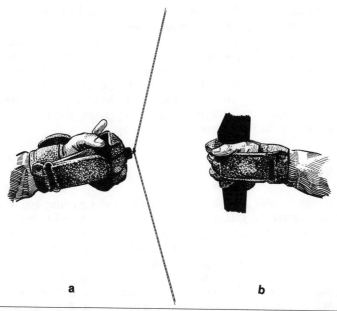

Figure 5.   Adapted archery devices developed by Applied Technology for Independent Living in cooperation with The Courage Center of Golden Valley, Minnesota: release cuff (a) and bow cuff (b).

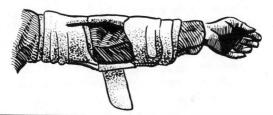

Figure 6.   Elbow support used with some hemiplegic archers and originally developed for spinal cord injured quadraplegics.

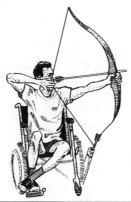

Figure 7.   Traditional alignment for a wheelchair archer with good upper body control.

The next step is to find the proper body position in the wheelchair and, again, to always be consistent. Find the location that gives you the maximum amount of balance. Move your hips forward or sag the upholstery in the back of your wheelchair. This may help with balance. A word of caution for wheelchair archers with good back balance—always relax against the chair back and never shoot while sitting up straight. Resting against the back of your wheelchair will provide more consistency to your technique. It should act as one of several reference points in your shooting style. After a few practice sessions, you will find the ideal position for your wheelchair and body.

Training

A part of each training session should be devoted to stretching and warm-up in order to avoid soreness, stiffness, and/or injury. Arm and wrist circles, shoulder shrugs, and stretching of a heavy rubber rope or tire tube are some quick exercises that will help to get the blood flowing to muscles of the arms and shoulders and thus improve your shooting performance.

These same exercises done immediately following a practice session will also help to prevent any soreness you might experience the day after shooting.

A general overall suggestion for training is to begin slowly. If you have chosen archery as a sport (whether it be for recreation or competition) you need to invest the time to learn archery correctly. During the initial states of training or learning the sport of archery, participants should not be worried about scoring large amounts of points. Emphasis needs to be placed on the development of proper technique. The key to effective training and practice is to correct each mistake as it occurs; uncorrected mistakes are more difficult to change over a period of time.

Begin by shooting at short distances. This will allow you to concentrate on proper form while ensuring an element of success. As skills and confidence increase, so then should the distance between archer and the target.

Archery is a very simple sport. Broken down into its simplest components, it involves six steps; positioning, nocking, drawing, holding, releasing, and fol-

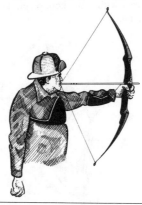

Figure 8. A stroke patient, paralyzed on the right side, uses a specially made mouthpiece to draw the bowstring.

lowing through. It is the consistent and accurate blending of these six tasks into one complete motion that requires a great deal of practice. Individual technique will change from archer to archer (compare Figure 1 to Figure 8), especially in programs where the participants have physical disabilities. However, the principle of shooting should never change. Consistency and accuracy remain the name of the game.

Those archers who have developed a good shooting base and have decided that competitive shooting is their next step must begin to consider archery as a sport that should be practiced every day. The skill and precision needed to be successful is something that is not acquired by picking up a bow only once a week. A great deal of time is needed to perfect the consistency and accuracy of a good competitive archer. If you decide to make the commitment, the time will certainly be well spent.

Safety and Protocol

The bow and arrow was at one time used as a weapon of war. It still remains a deadly weapon. Safety should be of prime concern to archers, coaches, and program supervisors. The Ontario Wheelchair Sports Association lists the following safety considerations in their *Introduction to Archery and Riflery Manual*.

1. Never draw and release a bow without an arrow in it, as this could break the bow and injure you.
2. Do not use someone else's equipment without their permission.
3. Never shoot an arrow while someone is on the target range. You can never assume an accurate release of the arrow.
4. Do not shoot an arrow straight up into the air. It could come down and hit you or someone close to you.
5. Keep the shooting range clear of anything that could cause a loose arrow to deflect.
6. Always wear an arm guard to protect yourself from the bow string.
7. Always keep the nocked arrow and bow pointed down the range toward the targets.
8. Make sure that your shooting range is secure at all entrances so that unexpected individuals are unable to enter the shooting area.
9. Never point or shoot at anything you do not intend to hit.
10. Use common sense and courtesy on the range at all times, and be alert to possibly dangerous situations (p. 3).

Note

For more information on wrist and arm supports, contact: Lyn Rourke, Courage Center, 3915 Golden Valley Road, Golden Valley, MN 55422, (612) 588-0811 or Dean Hughes, Applied Technology for Independent Living, 4732 Nevada Avenue, N., Crystal, MN 55428, (612) 537-6377. For additional information on archery contact: National Archery Association of the United States, 1750 East Boulder Street, Colorado Springs, CO 80909-5778, (303) 578-4576.

Additional Readings

Hagel, S. (1982, February). Quad archers. *Sports 'N Spokes,* pp. 16–17.

Heer, M. (1984, July/August). Elements of archery: Part 1—Getting started. *Sports 'N Spokes,* pp. 17–19.

Ontario Wheelchair Sports Association. (1981). *Introduction to archery and riflery.* Toronto: Ontario Wheelchair Sports Association.

Rourke, L. (1985, March/April). Elements of archery: Part III—Instruction. *Sports 'N Spokes,* pp. 18–19.

Rourke, L., & Heer, M. (1985, January/February). Elements of archery: Part II— equipment. *Sports 'N Spokes,* pp. 11–13.

Whitman, J. (1976, January/February). Archery—The silent sport. *Sports 'N Spokes,* pp. 14–16.

Rifle Shooting Tips

Gerry Dausman

In many competitive sports, physical advantage plays a big part. For example, football players tend to be big, jockeys are usually small, and basketball players are generally tall. In competitive target shooting, however, there are no physical advantages; anyone can compete successfully. What is most important to shooting is an understanding of basic fundamentals of marksmanship. These fundamentals are the same for a beginning shooter and an Olympic champion. The major difference between a beginner and an Olympic champion is the amount of time spent practicing those fundamentals.

This chapter will do three things. First, it will introduce you to shooting safety and fundamentals. Second, it will tell you a little about how they can be applied. Third, it will let you know where to get more information.

Safety

When handling air guns, the most important consideration for a shooter or instructor to be concerned with is safety. An air rifle, though not as powerful as a .22 rifle, can still be dangerous if improperly handled. Several safety rules should be kept in mind:

- Always keep the BB or air rifle pointed downrange in a safe direction.
- Treat every air rifle as if it were loaded.
- Be sure of your target and what is beyond.
- Obey all firing line commands.
- Keep your finger off the trigger until you are ready to fire.

Good Position

The first fundamental, a good shooting position, is simply holding the rifle steadily so that a shot may be fired accurately. Proper support and balance are the keys to holding the rifle steadily.

For proper support, the rifle should be held up by your bone structure as much as possible. This results in being able to hold your rifle steadier and for longer periods of time because you are tiring your muscles less.

Balance simply means adjusting your position so that you minimize the use of your muscles. A simple test to check your position is to relax your muscles. If you then start to fall over, you know you weren't properly balanced. You can shoot steadier and longer in a balanced position because you are not using your muscles to keep from falling over.

Remember the following tips on prone and wheelchair sitting (see also Figure 1):

- Both elbows on lapboard or table
- Left elbow slightly left of rifle
- Left hand near midpoint of rifle
- Head erect
- Butt of rifle firm in shoulder
- Body angled 10 to 20° off line of rifle
- Weight of upper body on elbows
- Weight of rifle on left elbow
- Legs relaxed
- Back relaxed

Sight Alignment

Sights are nothing more than convenient markers to show where the barrel is pointed. When you line the sights up on the targets, there are three things that you must watch: the front sight, the rear sight, and the target. Center the front sight in the rear sight, and at the same time, line the target up with the front sight.

The sights should be adjusted if your shots are all in one group but not at the center of the target. You should also adjust your sights when you start shooting at a different distance.

Trigger Squeeze

Once you have a position and good sight alignment, you want to squeeze the trigger. When squeezing the trigger, you do not want to disturb the alignment of the sights on the target. If you "pull" the trigger you will also pull the sights off the target. Squeezing the trigger should be done carefully, as carefully as if you were trying to squeeze just one drop out of an eyedropper.

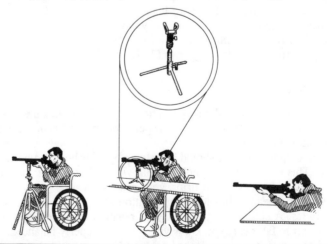

Figure 1. Shooting positions and rifle support allowed in CP—ISRA international competition. Coaches and shooters should refer to USCPAA rules for specifics on national competition.

Follow-Through

Just as a golfer or tennis player needs to follow through when completing a swing, a rifle shooter needs to follow through when completing a shot. Follow-through is simply keeping the sights lined up on the target for at least 1 full second after the shot is fired. This ensures that the sights stay well aligned as the pellet travels down the barrel.

Rifle Shooting Programs

The national governing body for shooting is the National Rifle Association. The NRA cosponsors and promotes several excellent programs nationwide in hopes of assisting individuals to develop both an appreciation for air guns and the proper skills to use them. These programs are listed in Table 1.

Table 1   Shooting Programs and Resources

Program	Resources
College Programs	NRA Collegiate Activities Department
NRA—Club Affiliation	NRA Clubs and Associations Department
Disabled Shooting Programs	Individual COSD member
Scouting Programs	Boy Scouts of America 1325 Walnut Hill Lane Irving, TX 75038-3096
NRA Junior Olympic Shooting Program	NRA Competition Division
4-H Shooting Sports Program	NRA Education and Training Division
Daisy and U.S. Jaycee Shooting Programs	U.S. Jaycee Headquarters P.O. Box 7 Tulsa, OK 74121
	Daisy Manufacturing Co., Inc. Rogers, AZ 72756
Explorer Scout and Crosman Air Gun Programs	Explorer Division of Boy Scouts of America 1325 Walnut Hill Lane Irving, TX 75038-3096
National Guard Four-Position Air Rifle Program	Unit Marksmanship Support Center Attn: Youth Programs P.O. Box 17267 Nashville, TN 37217-0267
Shooting Coach Certification Program	NRA Marksmanship Training Department, Education and Training Division

Equipment

Matching equipment to each competitor's functional ability is an important consideration in shooting. Several types of air guns are shown in Figure 2. An example of an air gun range and air gun targets are shown in Figure 3.

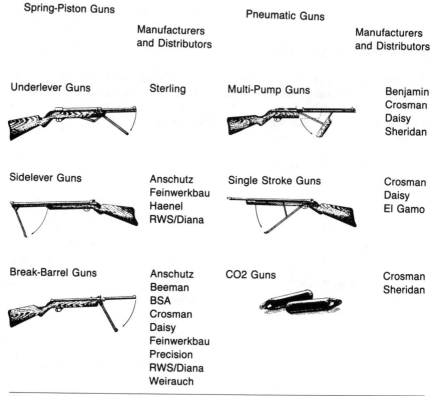

Spring-Piston Guns

Manufacturers and Distributors

Pneumatic Guns

Manufacturers and Distributors

| Underlever Guns | Sterling | Multi-Pump Guns | Benjamin Crosman Daisy Sheridan |

| Sidelever Guns | Anschutz Feinwerkbau Haenel RWS/Diana | Single Stroke Guns | Crosman Daisy El Gamo |

| Break-Barrel Guns | Anschutz Beeman BSA Crosman Daisy Feinwerkbau Precision RWS/Diana Weirauch | CO2 Guns | Crosman Sheridan |

Figure 2.   Types of air guns. *Note.*   Adapted from National Rifle Association (1984).

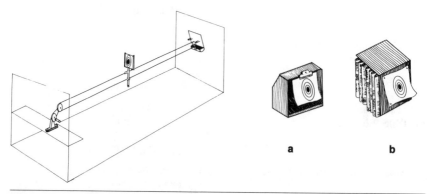

a   b

Figure 3.   An air gun range and inexpensive metal pellet trap target (a) and a trap target made from a cardboard box stuffed with newspapers (b).

Source List of Air Rifles and Air Pistols in the U.S.

Table 2 cites some of the major companies that manufacture and/or distribute air rifles and air pistols in the United States. Write these companies for their catalogs and program brochures. There are, of course, other distributors and brands not listed here. Check local gun shops, sporting goods dealers, and gun magazines for information on additional suppliers of air guns.

Table 2   U.S. Manufacturers and Distributors of Air Guns

Company	Air guns	Pellets
Beeman's Precision Arms, Inc.[a] 47 Paul Drive San Rafael, CA 94903 415/472-7121	Beeman FAS Feinwerkbau Webley Weirauch Wischo	Beeman Benjamin H/N RWS Sheridan
Benjamin Air Rifle Co.[a] 3205 Sheridan Road Racine, WI 53403 414/633-5424	Benjamin	Benjamin
Crosman Air Guns, Inc.[a,b] 980 Turk Hill Road Fairport, NY 14450 716/657-6161	Crosman RWS	Crosman
Daisy Manufacturing Co., Inc.[a,b] Rogers, AR 72756 501/636-1200	Daisy El Gamo	Daisy
Dynamit Nobel of America, Inc.[b] 105 Stonehurst Court Northvale, NJ 07647 201/767-1660	RWS/Diana	RWS
G.B. International[b] P.O. Box 16146 Cleveland, OH 44116 216/331-7991	Haenel	

(Cont.)

Table 2 (Cont.)

Company	Air guns	Pellets
Interarms, Ltd.[b] 10 Prince Street Alexandria, VA 22313 703/548-1400	Walther	
Marksman Products[a,b] 2133 Dominiques Street Torrance, CA 90509 213/320-8004	Marksman	Marksman
Precise International[b] 3 Chestnut Street Suffern, NY 10901 914/357-6200	Precise	Precise
Precision Sports, Inc.[b] P.O. Box 219 Ithaca, NY 14850 607/273-2993	BSA	BSA
Precision Sports International, Inc.[b] P.O. Box 1776 Westfield, MA 01086 413/562-5055	Anschutz	
Sheridan Products[a] 3205 Sheridan Road Racine, WI 53403 414/554-7900	Sheridan	Sheridan
Sterling Air Rifle[a] 3205 Sheridan Road Racine, WI 53403 414/633-5424	Sterling	Sterling

Note. List was obtained from NRA *Air Gun Shooting Manual.*
[a]Manufacturer. [b]Distributor.

Note

1. For more information, contact: NRA, 1600 Rhode Island Avenue, N.W., Washington, DC 20036 or NRA Shooting Sports Director, United States Olympic Training Center, 1776 East Boulder Street, Colorado Springs, CO 80909.

Additional Readings

Rifle Shooting
Basic Smallbore Rifle Guide. (No date). Fort Benning, GA: U.S. Army Marksmanship Unit.
Hickey, B. (1979). *Mental training*. Eagle River, AK: Totem Shooters Supplies.
International Rifle Marksmanship Guide. (1980). Fort Benning, GA: U.S. Army Marksmanship Unit.
Klingner, B. (1980). *Rifle shooting as a sport*. London: A.S. Barnes.
Klingner, B. (1981). *Rifle shooting: Training and competitions*. London: A.S. Barnes.
Pullum, B., & Hanenkrat, F.T. (1973). *Position rifle shooting*. NY: Winchester Press.
Pullum, B., & Hanenkrat, F.T. (1981). *Successful shooting*. Washington, DC: National Rifle Association.
National Rifle Association. (1984). *Air Gun Shooting*. Washington, DC: Author.
National Rifle Association. (1982). *Basic Rifle Marksmanship*. Washington, DC: Author.
National Rifle Association (1983). *The NRA Junior Rifle Handbook*. Washington, DC: Author.

Handgun Shooting
Antal, L. (1983). *Competitive pistol shooting*. Wakefield, England: EP Publishing.
Chandler, J. (1983). *The target gun book of pistol coaching*. Droitwich, England: Peterson.
Pistol Marksmanship Guide. (No date). Fort Benning, GA: U.S. Army Marksmanship Unit.
Standl, H. (1977). *Pistol shooting*. Toronto: Coles.

General Books on Shooting
The marksmanship instructors and coaches manual. (1971). Fort Benning, GA: U.S. Army Marksmanship Training Unit.
Profiles of a champion. (1974). Fort Benning, GA: U.S. Army Marksmanship Unit.

Swimming to Win

Libby Anderson

Swimming is an activity that many look at as enjoyable, relaxing, and stress-reducing. But to the competitive swimmer and his or her coach, swimming involves a lot more. To become efficient, each swimmer needs to be aware of many things, such as the laws of physics, safety considerations, physical abilities, training specifics, and balance, buoyancy, and propulsion through the water. The best place to start is with an understanding of the effect of water on the body.

Balance

Balance should be examined in four quadrants. The center of gravity and the center of buoyancy must be dealt with by dividing the body into four parts; two parts being above and below the waist, and two additional parts being the right and left sides of the body. As one part of the body, for example, the arm, is being moved, it affects the balance of the other parts. Poor balance can affect body roll, timing of the breath, and coordination of the stroke.

Buoyancy

Buoyancy deals with the force of water that supports each body segment in a horizontal position. Gravity pushes down on each body segment. Some body segments are more buoyant than others, depending on how much fat they contain (the greater the percentage of fat, the more buoyant). The buoyant effect of water is modified as the arms or legs move through the skill pattern. When an arm is recovered above the water, this affects the buoyancy of the rest of the body.

Propulsion

Propulsion is forward movement through the water. It is affected by the swimmer's physical abilities and by the effect of the movement on the swimmer's balance and buoyancy. As the swimmer moves through the water, he or she should be working on reducing resistance to that movement—for example, by avoiding the head being too low in the water, improper entry of the hands, or movement in an up and down motion. The trade-off is an increase in the propulsion force necessary to overcome the body's slowing down due to the increase in resistance.

Another factor affecting propulsion is Newton's law of action and reaction, which simply states that for every action, there is an equal and an opposite reaction. In swimming, this is the force directed away from the desired line of travel. If the swimmer's hand enters the water by pushing down, the response will be an up and down movement in the body position. If the swimmer's free-style pull is wide or overreaches, the body position will move from side to side. To be efficient, force should be directed backward in the line of travel.

These three areas combined can work for or against a swimmer. Stroke drills, adapted strokes, workouts, and flotation devices can improve a swimmer's balance, buoyancy, and propulsion and can make him a more efficient and faster swimmer.

Stroke Work

The key to efficiency in performing the four competitive strokes is in the adaptation of the stroke to the person's abilities. Assessment of a swimmer's abilities can be done by evaluating the effect of the disability on the land and in the water. How do they walk and balance themselves? How much range of motion do they have? How has the disability affected their coordination and what kind of arm strength do they have?

When in the water, break each stroke into five parts: entry, catch, pull, push, and recovery. Follow the swimmer through each phase. Check to see how balance and stroke technique are affected, how buoyancy is affected by his or her spasticity or contractures, and how the swimmer turns to take a breath. Be sure to note the effect on body position as the swimmer moves through the water.

As the swimmer performs each stroke, develop a checklist in order to concentrate on the specifics of each stroke.

- Hand position—How is the hand positioned during the entry, pull, and exit? What is the position of the hand in relation to the elbow and the shoulder?
- Elbow position—Is the elbow in a bent position? Does it slide through the stroke, or is it used during the positive phase? Where is the elbow in relation to the body during the entry, pull, and exit?
- Line of pull—With any stroke, it is important that as your hand(s) move through the water the movement be efficient. Check the length of the pull, its width, and its pattern. Is it a straight or a bending pull? Make sure you know where the power or the strongest point is.
- Body roll—Balance is directly affected by the arm stroke and timing of the kick. For every action, there is an equal reaction. Body roll adjusts for stroke recovery and depth of pull. Watch for imbalances in muscle strength and flexibility.
- Timing of kick/pull—Most kicking is to enhance arm action (except for the breaststroke). Watch timing to be sure kicking occurs at the most effective point. Adjustment of kick during the fly can greatly assist with breathing.
- Ankle, knee, and hip flexibility—Flexibility will affect the direction of the kick and can cause drag that will produce an improper kick. Recovery of the legs will affect body position and forward movement. Remember action versus reaction.
- Breathing—Timing of the breath to the stroke varies with each disability. Breathing should occur during the push phase of the stroke, but some disa-

bilities shorten the length of the push. Modify the stroke and/or the timing to meet this need.

After determining which part of the stroke you want to work on, be sure *to work on one detail at a time*. Repeat this one often until it becomes automatic before introducing another detail. Make sure the swimmer understands your directions. Have the swimmer repeat and discuss with you why he or she should be pulling in a certain manner. Use the same cues in practice, and don't be too picky. Distinguish between what is important and what is not. Encourage your swimmers to practice at home. For example, have them practice arm patterns while lying in bed or sitting in their wheelchairs. Always keep in mind their individuality and your ability to adapt the stroke to their needs.

Stroke Drills

All strokes can be divided into the five parts discussed earlier: entry, catch, pull, push, and recovery. Stroke drills are repetitive drills that work on one particular part of a stroke. For example, the double-arm backstroke drill works on the recovery and the entry of the little finger. Listed next are some examples of drills for the freestyle and the butterfly. Using your own swimmers, you can further expand the number of drills and by using funny names, expand your swimmers' awareness of the water and how to use it.

1. Freestyle
   Drills for pull
   - Dogpaddle with underwater recovery.
   - Rope drill—Straddle a rope or garden hose and pull yourself up the rope.
   - Kickboard drill—Right arm only; hold board with left hand.
   - Tarzan—Heads-up freestyle; concentrate on short entry and short pull.
   - Finger drag—High elbow recovery; keep fingertips in the water.
   - Teepee drill—High elbow recovery.
   Drills for entry
   - Fist swim—Swim with fist to eliminate hands on entry.
   - Doughnut drill—Encourages shoulder width entry.
   Drills for body position
   - Chicken free—Thumbs in armpits, swimmer swims rolling body and accentuating the shoulder roll.
   - Kick with board.
   - Kick with swim fins.
   - Corkscrew kick—Kick six kicks on the front, right side, back, and left side, and continue to kick as body position changes.
   - Kick with tennis shoes and fins.
   Drills for breathing
   - Dog paddle—Breathing forward.
   - Dog paddle—Breathing sideways.
   - Twinkle—Draw a twinkle star on the bend of the elbow of the breathing arm. Directions are to follow the twinkle, breathe, and beat it back by putting the face into the water before the elbow comes around.

2. Butterfly
   Drill for pull
   - Dogfly—Dog paddle, but with both arms performing the butterfly stroke, and recovering underwater.

   Drill for recovery
   - Slidefly—Similar to the finger drag, but arms recover sliding across the top to the water.

   Drills for timing
   - Four-kick fly—Four kicks to one fly pull works on timing of the second kick.
   - One-arm fly—Right or left arm only is timed to fly kick; kick as the hand enters and kick as the hand finishes.
   - Free with fly—Freestyle arms times to the fly kick.

   Drills for kick
   - Kick—Without board, breaststroke arm to breathe.
   - Side kick—Kick on side, breathe with freestyle arm stroke.

Teaching Techniques

Sometimes water and the CP athlete don't mix very well. For some reason the athlete can't control his breathing well enough, spasticity overaccentuates movements, and lack of fat makes forward movement difficult. All this may seem impossible to deal with, but there are ways to overcome these obstacles.

Stroke Skill Development

First, work with what the swimmer *can* do. If he or she is a backstroker, let the swimmer experience that success. Many times, backstroke distance workouts can lead to endurance and the ability to bob and control breathing for swimming on the front. Turning over from back to front and front to back can lead to an efficient form of breathing for many Class I and Class II athletes.

Next, deal with what their physical abilities will allow them to do. Your swimmer may not be able to reach over his or her body to turn over, but he or she might be able to use the shoulder or elbow to initiate that rollover. Couple the elbow with a head movement, add a leg that crosses over the midline at the hips, and you've started the swimmer controlling his or her own turnover.

Many swimmers are limited in their shoulder movements. The swimmers should be taught how to fin on their back, and breaststroke on their front. Symmetrical movements allow for better balance in the water. Recovery under the water maintains a horizontal body position. As the swimmer develops better control over his or her body in the water, add an above-the-water recovery on the back and develop a double-arm backstroke. Or, modify the breaststroke into a long dog paddle pull and use the body roll to take a breath. Practicing the breathing techniques before the introduction of the new strokes will better prepare the swimmer for the change in complexity of the stroke.

To increase understanding of stroke patterns, use equipment available at the pool. Lie over the lane line and practice the breaststroke arm pull. With the lane line at their chests, the swimmers get immediate tactile feedback as they pull their arms level to their shoulders. Use the lane line for backstroke pull drills. Tell the swimmers to reach back and grab the lane line and pull themselves past their hand. The grabbing and pulling will be reinforced as they feel the movement. All teaching should include as many of the learning modes—visual, auditory, and tactile—as possible. By using funny words to point out improper skills, the same cue words in practice, and crazy names for stroke drills, swimmers will learn quickly whether to float or not.

Flotation Devices

Initially, all movements should be kept slow and simple. Lots of practice and learning the gross motor movements will serve as an introduction to the more difficult skill of putting kick, pull, and breath together. Many swimmers will need something more consistent—a flotation device.

A flotation device should be used when a swimmer needs this kind of consistent support; for example, water wings. With a water wing on each arm, the swimmer can concentrate on the action he or she is trying to perform. When the swimmer can consistently perform the skill, dependence on the device should be reduced to the point where it is no longer needed or is needed only minimally. But if a swimmer needs, for example, head support because of lack of control, then they should use a flotation device, for example, a float collar, at all times. The question is what is appropriate and when is it needed.

Flotation devices are useful when teaching new skills or when concentrating on one particular skill; for example, using a pull buoy. Before teaching the backstroke, a swimmer with balance problems might use a flotation device at first to ease fears and increase endurance; later, it would be taken away as the swimmer becomes more proficient. Inner tubes are useful for a swimmer who is trying to swim in a horizontal position. A flotation device is effective for a swimmer during the backstroke but limits breathing during the freestyle.

Flotation devices should be chosen with a number of criteria in mind including uneven muscle development, joint flexibility, spasticity, head control, amount of lean body mass, and the skill level of the individual swimmer. Experience in the water can be a major determining factor. As the efficiency of a swimmer increases, a different type of flotation device will be needed. By having a wide selection of flotation devices, based on a continuum of need each swimmer can be assured of getting the right amount of flotation he or she needs to develop the most efficient swim stroke.

The floats vary in size and the amount of support they give the swimmer. A practical approach to this problem is on a continuum of need that begins with total dependence and moves up to complete independence. For more information on flotation devices, refer to the next chapter of this manual.

Conclusion

Experience will be the key to a successful swim program. With an understanding of the effect of the disability on the water, stroke drills and modifications, teaching techniques and flotation devices, your swimmers will become proficient in their swim strokes and gain from the experience.

Additional Readings

American National Red Cross. (1977). *Adapted aquatics*. Washington, DC: American National Red Cross.

American National Red Cross. (1977). *Methods in adapted aquatics: A manual for the instructor* (pp. 13-14). Washington, DC: American National Red Cross.

American National Red Cross. (1981). *Swimming and aquatic safety*. Washington, DC: American National Red Cross.

Bradley, N.A., Fuller, J.L., Pozoa, R.S. , & Willmers, L.E. (1981, May/June). PFD's. *Sports 'N Spokes,* pp. 23-25.

Counsilman, J. E. (1968). *The science of swimming*. Englewood Cliffs, NJ: Prentice-Hall.

Counsilman, J. E. (1977). *Competitive swimming manual: For coaches and swimmers*. Bloomington, IN: Counsilman Co.

Maglischo, E.W. (1982). *Swimming faster*. Palo Alto, CA: Mayfield Publishing.

United States Swimming. (1985). *Handbook for adapted competitive swimming*. 1750 East Boulder St., Colorado Springs, CO 80907

To Float or Not to Float

Jeffery A. Jones

An essential factor contributing to a coach's ability to successfully run a swim program for individuals with cerebral palsy (CP) and other physical disabilities will be their knowledge and use of flotation devices. In respect to CP sports, there has been and will continue to be some debate over the issue of an athlete being a true competitive athlete when using or not using a flotation device. The United States Cerebral Palsy Athletic Association (USCPAA) established rules allowing the use of floats in competition by Class I and Class II athletes only. However, regardless of one's opinion as to the legitimacy of floats for competition, it is obvious that many individuals with CP require the use of flotation devices in order to swim or while becoming more proficient in a given swimming stroke. Because most swim programs for the disabled are usually not run exclusively for competitive swimmers, the need for floats within your program is very likely.

When operating your swim program, you will find that for a number of reasons many individuals with CP (especially those with more involved disabilities) are not great floaters. Because many also do not have the ability to coordinate their extremities to the point of keeping themselves above water, the use of a float for swimming is the logical solution. Usually it is not very difficult to convince a swimmer who truly needs a float to use one. Problems may arise, however, with traumatic brain-injured swimmers (TBI, or closed head-injured), especially if the individual was recently injured or swam before his or her accident. Individuals in this situation may not realize the extent of their disability. Because they never needed a float before, they may be apprehensive about using one now. A *very* closely supervised attempt to swim without a float will usually illustrate to them that, although awkward at first, a flotation device, at least at this time, is a most essential item.

Beginning swimmers should be given a swimming test while being closely supervised and evaluated in terms of their need for a float. Usually, if a swimmer is able to swim two lengths (50 m) without stopping to rest, he or she is competent to swim without a float. However, lifeguards should be made aware of who is a "strong" swimmer and who is not. Remember, not all individuals with disabilities will require a float in order to swim. Also, some of your weaker swimmers will be capable of swimming in the shallow end of the pool without a float, where security is easily gained by standing up. A float in this case would only be used for endurance training when the swimmer attempts swimming repetitive laps. If your swim program involves both strong and weak competitive and noncompetitive swimmers, you should consider dividing the pool into different workout areas, using lane lines. Distinctly separate areas should be provided for swimmers wishing to swim repetitive laps, and those who, because of poor swimming skills, need to be restricted to the shallow end of the pool.

The security provided by the float to a swimmer cannot be overemphasized. It is very important that each float fit correctly and that each float is put on and secured properly every time. When operating a large program, properly fitting floats on swimmers will usually take up a large portion of your swim time. Schedule around it. Arrive early prior to pool time and take the time to do it right. There is nothing more frightening to a swimmer or pool staff than a swimmer's head falling through a loose-fitting float. Take the time. Floats can also loosen during the course of a swim session. Coaches and lifeguards should make an effort to check all floats on a regular basis throughout the swim period.

Fitting a float to a swimmer is as important to a swimmer as a properly fitting wheelchair is to a track athlete, not only in terms of safety, but also for the opportunity to develop the most efficient swimming stroke possible. The most popular flotation device used today is the U.S. Coast Guard–approved Type II personal flotation device (PFD) (see Figure 1). There are several types on the market, all designed and tested according to Coast Guard guidelines, based on average *able-bodied* male swimmers. Depending on the nature of your swimmer's disability, a Type II PFD (or any U.S. Coast Guard–approved PFD) may or may not be appropriate. Coaches should be aware that there are a number of suitable alternatives.

The following list presents various flotation devices in an order showing progression from total dependency to swimming independently:

- Danmar sectional raft
- PFD with head support
- Delta swim system
- Waist belt
- Waist bubble
- Head float
- Water wings
- No float; independent swimming

Floats vary in size from small water wings (Figure 4) or limb floats to the multipiece Danmar body support float (Figure 2) or the Delta Float System (Figure 3), which can be pieced together to custom fit your swimmer.

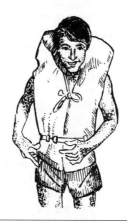

Figure 1. U.S. Coast Guard-approved Type II PFD.

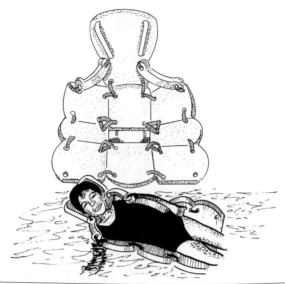

Figure 2.   A Danmar sectional raft.

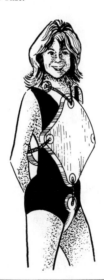

Figure 3.   The Delta float system.

Tire tubes, Styrofoam bubbles, inflatable collars, water ski waist belts, PFDs, life vests, and jackets have all been used in swim programs for the disabled. There are also a number of specially made multipurpose swim rings and head floats that allow instructors the freedom to work with the swimmer's arms and legs, as well as floats that compensate for lateral rotation due to uneven muscle development (see Figure 5).

When deciding what type of float your swimmer will need, you need to take several factors into consideration. The individual's swimming ability (dictated

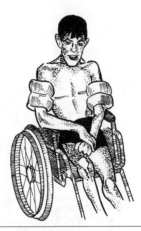

Figure 4.   Water wings.

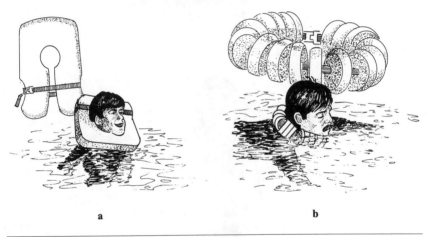

a   b

Figure 5.   Danmar head float (a) and swim rings (b).

by physical strength, flexibility, and buoyancy), his or her swimming style or technique, the swimmer's experience in the water, and any related disabilities (i.e., seizures) should all be evaluated when choosing a float. You may have 20 swimmers in your program, each requiring a different type of float. The float that works for one Class II may not be appropriate for another. Some Class II swimmers will swim in a vertical position using a tire tube or circular float, whereas others will be more efficient swimming in a supine position with or without a float (see Figure 6). A hemiplegic Class III will most likely require a different float than a beginning Class IV swimmer.

A swimmer's need or dependence on a float may change as a swimmer gains confidence, strength, and skill in a particular swimming stroke. The bulky PFD is often replaced by streamlined waist belts or waist bubbles, which in time may even be replaced by water wings. It should be noted, however, that there are no clear-cut prerequisites like time spent in a program or number of seconds cut

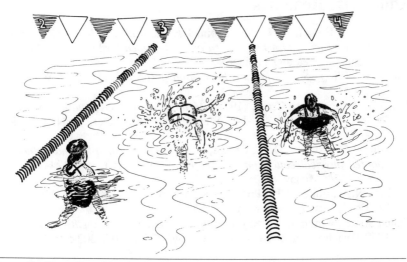

Figure 6.   Two Class II swimmers using different flotation devices in competition.

off a personal record that dictate when a swimmer will progress from one float to another float, or discontinue the use of a float altogether. Progression to independent swimming (if it happens at all) will be as individual as the initial selection of a float.

Coaches and athletes should remember that a float, no matter what kind, is no substitute for an athlete's familiarity with the water and a staff's lifeguarding responsibility. If the swimmer has the ability, he or she should become as proficient as possible in treading water, in righting skills from horizontal to vertical and supine to prone, and in holding his or her breath under water. In respect to lifeguarding, the staff should not treat each swimmer identically. Problems and accidents can and have happened to swimmers with and without floating devices, in good conditions, and with years of swimming experience. So, be careful. Do not compromise your program and the safety of your swimmers with poor lifeguarding practices.

It is difficult to collect in a few pages all there is to know about flotation devices, the characteristics of the swimmers that need them, and the progression in which they should be used. Experience will be your best teacher. Do not limit your ability by reducing your options. The fact that USCPAA restricts the use of floats to Class I and II swimmers in competition should not prevent you from using them with other swimmers. If your program follows the norm, it will have a wide variety of swimmers, including recreational swimmers, athletes looking for an alternative to their daily training schedule, and competitive swimmers, all of different classes, swimming styles, and swimming experience. The key is experience, for there is no better teacher than experience.

Note

For more information concerning the latest in personal flotation devices and other swim aids, contact: Danmar Products, Inc., 2390 Winewood, Ann Arbor, MI 48102, (313) 761-1990.

Additional Readings

Adams, R.C., Daniel, A.N., McCabbin, J.A., & Rullman, L. (1982). *Games, sports and exercise for the physically handicapped* (3rd ed., pp. 339–358). Philadelphia: Lea and Febiger.

Allen, A. (1981). *Sports for the handicapped* (pp. 41-43). NY: Waler and Company.

American National Red Cross. (1977). *Methods in adapted aquatics: A manual for the instructor* (pp. 13–14). Washington, DC: American National Red Cross.

Arnhem, D.D., Auxter, D., & Crowe, W.C. (1977). *Principles and methods of adapted physical education and recreation.* (3rd ed.), (pp. 124–128). St. Louis: C.V. Mosby.

Bradley, N.A., Fuller, J.L., Pozos, R.S., & Willmers, L.E. (1981, May/June). PFD's. *Sports 'N Spokes,* pp. 23–25.

United States Swimming. (1985). *Handbook for adapted competitive swimming.* 1750 East Boulder St., Colorado Springs, CO 80707, 303-578-4578

Wheelchair Boccia

Jeffery A. Jones

An indoor version of the Italian game of lawn bowling, boccia represents one of the most challenging and fastest growing sports offered to cerebral palsy (CP) athletes. Whether it be individual boccia (one against one) or team boccia (three against three), this game involves a tremendous amount of skill, precision, and strategy, which requires a great deal of practice in order to be competitive.[1]

This chapter will discuss the generalities of the game of boccia with specific emphasis on the court, player positioning, player technique, the role of the captain, and game strategies.

The Court

A boccia court consists of two areas, the player's boxes and the playing area. The playing area also consists of two parts, the nonvalid target area and the valid target area (see Figure 1).

The players' boxes consist of six equal-sized boxes. Each player must stay completely within his or her own box during play. With the exception of the open

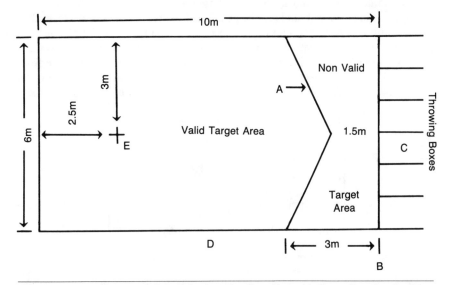

Figure 1. A = First throw line; B = throwing line; C = aide-lines; D = border lines; E = the cross.

173

end of the box, no part of the player, wheelchair, or ramp may touch outside the 1 m wide, 2 1/2-m long box.

The nonvalid target area (the smaller of two sections of the playing area), represents the area of the court that the target ball must exceed in order to be considered in play. If the target ball lands within this nonvalid target area, another player will have the opportunity to attempt placing the target ball within the valid playing area. This area is important to note when selecting your players' positions within the players' boxes. The shape of the nonvalid area allows a weaker player to get the ball in the valid area much more easily if he or she is placed in either the third or fourth box.

The valid target area makes up the remaining part of the playing area. Once the target ball has been placed in this area, the entire 10 m by 6 m court becomes the playing area. Remember, although the target ball must be within the valid area, points can be scored by any ball within the entire playing area, including the nonvalid area (see Figure 2).

A final important part of the playing area is the cross (Point E on Figure 1). If and when the target ball goes out-of-bounds, it is returned to the court and placed on the cross. This, of course, can be very advantageous if your team's balls are closer to the cross than your opponents. Strategy behind using the cross is discussed later in this article.

Player Positioning

When selecting the playing positions for your athletes, consider the athletes' overall playing ability (Figure 3). By placing stronger players on the outside boxes and placing the weaker players in the middle, a team is increasing the likelihood of having the target ball land in the valid target area.

Players using ramps should also be positioned in the outside boxes. Generally, with a ramp it is harder to control the speed of the ball for close shots, and the use of a ramp usually enables a player to reach all the points on the court as well.

A coin toss will determine which team gets to position their players in the first, third, and fifth or the second, fourth, and sixth boxes. During individual boccia games, the coin toss allows a player to select whatever box he or she wishes,

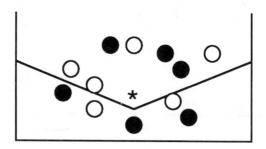

Figure 2.   Once target ball is placed in the valid area, points can be scored by balls regardless of their location.

ST/R	ST/R	W	W	ST/R	ST/R
1	2	3	4	5	6

Figure 3. Player position by athlete ability.

leaving one of the remaining five to the opponent. In most cases, players in individual boccia select the third and fourth boxes from which to play.

Selection of the player's position is one of many strategic maneuvers in boccia.
Remember, if your team starts the game, the opposing team will have the final
placement of the target ball. This may or may not be important; however, as
in baseball, many games are won during last at bats.

Technique

At the national and international levels, the game of boccia is currently open to
only Class I and Class II athletes. However, many programs across the country
use boccia as a recreational and/or competitive game for athletes of all classes.
For the purpose of this chapter, we will limit discussions to Class I and II.

Players have the choice of playing *with* or *without* an assistive device or chute
(see Figure 4). Competitions are divided into three divisions; Class I without
chutes, Class II without chutes, and Class I and II with chutes. Athletes should
spend time practicing with and without a chute before deciding which division
to compete in. Several factors should be considered, including the ability to grasp
the ball, the ability to release during throw motion, and the ability to place the
ball accurately on *all* areas of the playing court.

When determining the most efficient technique, one should not overlook the
lower extremities (see Figure 5). Many Class I and II athletes who have little
or no functional use of their hands possess remarkable foot coordination. Many
of these athletes will already be involved in Class II lower events, such as track
and/or the kicking field events.

As in many sports, adapted equipment allows many athletes to participate in
boccia who might otherwise be unable to or otherwise be noncompetitive. The
use of chutes or ramps is restricted to a single division in which both Class I
and II compete together, the assistive device being the equalizing factor. An athlete's ability to use a chute or ramp effectively depends on several factors, including the type of ramp release mechanism or technique used by the athlete and
the need for additional assistance. Figure 4 shows the most popular chute used
in competition. Made of plastic or aluminum pipe, it can be left whole or cut
down the middle. Figure 6 shows a more complicated device that includes a swiveling base, height adjustments that ultimately control speed and distance, and a
release lever.

The type and variety of chutes is only limited by the imagination of the builder.
One should always remember, however, that design must be primarily based on

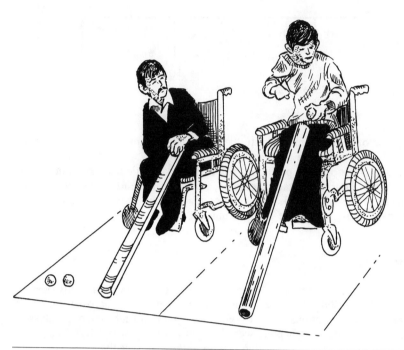

Figure 4. Players using assistive chutes.

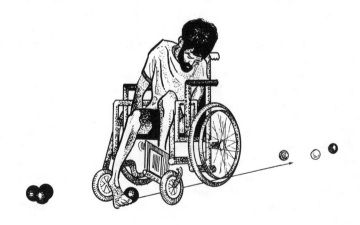

Figure 5. Athlete using lower extremity to play boccia.

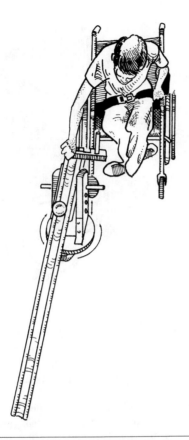

Figure 6.   A complex-style chute with a swiveling base.

the athlete's functional ability and that as in swimming, where one float may not be appropriate for different swimmers, a boccia ramp that is successful for one athlete may not be for another. Figure 7 shows a different version of the original ramp shown in Figure 6. Note the different solution to the same problem: efficient release of the ball.

Assisting the Athlete

Boccia rules do allow athletes to be assisted by a coach or an aide during competition. An important interpretation of this rule is the difference between assisting and coaching. Coaching is obviously not allowed. The primary need for assistance is usually preparation and placement of the ball prior to the athlete's delivery. The nature of a leather boccia ball is such that it can lose its roundness very easily, thus requiring a coach to reshape it before putting it back into play. This preparation is done to ensure the best possible roll of the ball. Coaches are also allowed

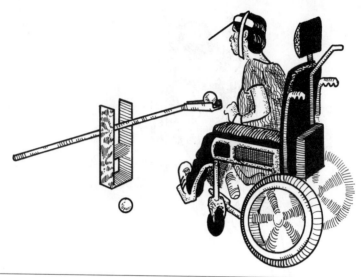

Figure 7.   A height-adjustable chute.

to place the ball either on the ramp or in the athlete's hand in order to assist the athlete in properly positioning the ball before releasing it either mechanically or manually. It is important to remember that the *athlete* must initiate the movement of the ball and that the coach or aide should only assist in the positioning of the ball.

The other major area of assistance is helping an athlete with his or her ramp or chute. Assistance may include changing its direction, changing its height, changing the chute's entire position within the throwing box, or even holding the chute for the athlete. The main rule clarification in respect to assistance with a chute is that once the game has begun, the person assisting the athlete must keep his or her back to the playing court and must make adjustment only after being asked by the athlete (see Figure 8). This is necessary to ensure that the athlete, not the coach, is actually initiating the changes. When working with athletes who are nonverbal, the coach must predetermine a method of communication, usually based on a series of questions from the coach to the athlete.

It is suggested that whatever system is established between an athlete and a coach, it should stay consistent. It will be difficult at best for an athlete to develop good technique if a major component of his or her game is constantly changing.

The Role of the Captain

Many times the success of a team in team boccia tournament depends heavily on the role of their team's captain. In boccia nothing happens unless it is initiated by one of the two captains.

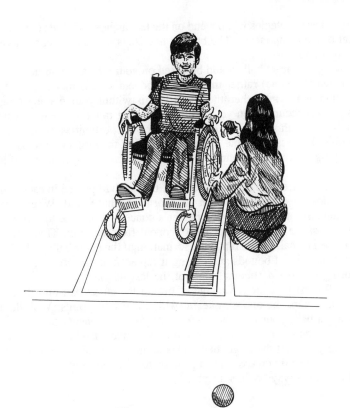

Figure 8.   An athlete receiving assistance fairly with his chute.

Captains are involved in the coin toss. They decide players' positions and select the order in which his or her team's players will play. The captain is the only person allowed to talk to the officials or other players during play (with the exception of an assistant's questions to a nonverbal player). The captain is virtually a player/coach. He or she must be knowledgeable of the rules and must know when to question officials. The captain must be aware at all times of the target ball's position, as well as be familiar with all his or her teammates' playing styles, abilities and limitations, and how they all relate to the position of the target ball.

Game Strategy

Whether it be individual or team boccia, placement of the target ball and the ensuing placement of game balls always involves a number of options and basic strategy. These strategies will depend on the techniques and skills of your players and that of their opponents. The bottom line stays the same: Score more points than your opponents.

Throwing the target ball should be based on your athlete's individual ''game'' (or your team's game) rather than your opponent's. It is much easier to battle for position and points when the target ball is within your playing range. The ideal situation occurs when your athlete's playing range is greater than that of the opponent. Each side has an equal number of opportunities to place the target ball in play. It is essential that during your round, the target ball remains within your playing range. As in tennis, it is important that a player score off his own serve.

Next to the placement of the target ball, the last ball played in each round can have the most significant effect on the scoring of that round. When faced with placing the last ball into play, the player's concern should be to score as many points as possible or to prevent the opponent from scoring. This can be done by using the last ball to rearrange the formation of the other balls or by knocking the target ball out-of-bounds and having it replaced on the cross, thus changing the scoring for that particular round at the last minute.

Figure 9 illustrates the advantage of hitting the target ball out-of-bounds. In the original setup, the opposing team (white) had four points. With the repositioned target ball, your team has two points, your opponents have none. In all, there is a six-point difference in the score. You may also be faced with a situation where you want the target ball knocked out-of-bounds to lessen your opponent's score, even if you are not in a position to score yourself. Remember, points earned are not always points scored.

Practice Makes Perfect

Not unlike many sports that require skill and precision, the better boccia players are usually those who spend lots of time practicing the game. Coaches and players must remember there are *two* parts to this game, the physical and the mental.

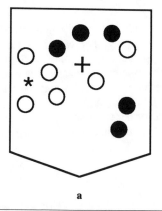
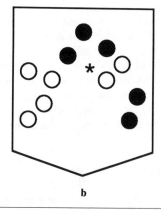

a   b

Figure 9.   Original setup (a) and relocated target ball (b). * = Target ball; O = Opposing team; ● = Home team.

The physical part involves the throwing, pushing, rolling, and/or releasing the ball. Time must be taken to discover and learn the most efficient way to place the ball into play and to reach as many parts of the court as possible. The more complicated the technique (i.e., an elaborate ramp), the more time that will be required.

A problem that confronts many athletes wanting to work on the physical part is facilities. Availability of an official-sized, hard, smooth, and level boccia court often prevents players from practicing the game as it was designed. Some suggestions for alternatives include gymnasiums, racquetball courts, school hallways, all-purpose rooms, cafeterias, basement floors, driveways, or any other place with a little room to roll the ball. Remember, the game includes two parts. The mental part of boccia, the what-to-do and what-not-to-do strategies, can be taught on a living room rug with marbles or even a kitchen table with marshmallows. If your program can't afford boccia sets for all your athletes, send them home with tennis balls or baseballs or anything with which they can simulate the game.

The key to successful boccia competition is never being faced with a game situation that your players haven't seen before. Practice at home supplemented by quality instruction and practice games during your formal practices should help your players prepare for whatever may happen come tournament day.

Conclusion

Boccia is a very easy game to learn, and, at the same time, it is very complicated, requiring skill and strategy in order to win. This chapter is simply an introduction to the game. It cannot replace the United States Cerebral Palsy Athletic Association (USCPAA) rules, for there are a number of specific regulations not covered within this chapter. Given enough time to learn all the rules, to practice team and individual strategies, and to incorporate adapted equipment if needed, boccia can be an enjoyable and successful event for anyone, both as a competitive sport and a recreational game.

Note

Boccia sets are available from: Newton Products, F.A.O., Mr. R. Skitt, Meadway Works, The Spastics Society, Garretts Green Lane, Birmingham, England, Tel: 021-783-6084; or Marienne W. Sorensen, Dansk Handicap Idraets-Forbund Idraettens HUS, Brandy Stadion, DK 2605 Brandy, Denmark

Additional Readings

Boccia. (1985, October). *Classification and sport rules manual* (4th ed., pp. 22–28). The Netherlands: CP-ISRA.

DeAngelis, R. (1980). Wheelchair boccia strategy. *Training guide to cerebral palsy sports* (2nd ed., pp. 90-93). NY: UCPA, Inc.

Bowling

Jerry McCole
Jamy Black McCole
James Patterson

Prior to the rise of the cerebral palsy (CP) sports movement in the 1970s, bowling was one of the few sports activities available to the person with CP.

Some might wish to take issue with the term "athlete" being applied to a bowler. It could be argued that competitive bowling does not require a person to train rigorously to the extent that certain track and field events do.

Putting discussions of terminology aside, there is little doubt that bowling depends on the coordination of muscular activity, a high degree of eye-hand coordination, concentration, and consistency. In this sense it can be compared to riflery, archery, and boccia. It also has the advantage of being adaptable to persons with virtually any degree of involvement and any disability.

We will focus on bowling in terms of specialized equipment requirements, coaching strategy, staffing needs and handicapping procedures.

Equipment

There are two basic types of bowlers: ambulatory and nonambulatory. With regard to equipment, the primary concern of the ambulatory bowler is to find a ball suited to his or her individual needs. The finger holes should be spaced so that the bowler can grip the ball firmly and comfortably. If the holes are too far apart, there may be difficulty in controlling the timing of the release of the ball. A premature release usually can be traced to an excessive spread of the fingers. Conversely, finger holes too close together will often lead to complaints of cramps in the center of the palm. In general, a bowler should choose the heaviest ball that allows complete control without leading to excessive fatigue.

For those bowlers who have difficulty handling a standard ball, balls with spring-loaded retractable handles are available. Also, some bowlers prefer to use a two-pronged ball pusher similar to the instruments used in shuffleboard (see Figure 1).

Nonambulatory bowlers have a wide variety of equipment and bowling methods available to them. Class V and VI athletes concerned about balance difficulties have the option of bowling in a standing position using assistive devices (i.e., crutch, walker, or chair), bowling free arm from a wheelchair or standard chair, or bowling from a wheelchair with a ramp (Figure 2). If a chair is used, the chair's legs should be equipped with soft rubber tips to avoid damaging the approach surface. Often Class IV bowlers, and at times strong Class III bowlers, choose to bowl free arm instead of using a ramp (Figure 3). Ramp bowlers have demon-

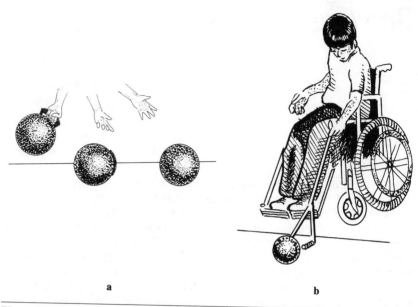

a   b

Figure 1. Spring-loaded handle balls provide an alternative to conventional bowling balls (a). A bowling stick or ball pusher can also be used by bowlers unable to throw a ball (b).

strated a high degree of success with various types of chutes or ramps made either of wood or tubular steel.

Five variables are to be considered in designing and building a usable bowling ramp:

1. The *ease* with which a bowler can approach and use the ramp from a standard wheelchair. Some bowlers prefer a ramp that attaches to the arms of a wheelchair (see Figure 4). Others prefer a free-standing ramp that can be moved independently of any movement of the bowler's wheelchair.
2. The *smoothness* with which the ramp delivers the ball to the lane surface.
3. The *weight* of the ramp. Because the forward momentum of the ball tends to force the ramp in the opposite direction, the ramp must either be secured in some way or be weighted to provide stability after the ball is released (see Figure 5).
4. *Portability.*
5. *Nonabrasiveness* of the base and legs of the ramp. The ramp should either have nonmarring surfaces on the points at which it touches the floor, or should be insulated from the approach surface by a pad (see Figure 6). Large scraps of carpeting make good cheap pads for this purpose.

In regard to the type of ball to be used with ramps, it has been our experience that plugged or undrilled balls (i.e., without holes) are highly desirable in that they allow a greater degree of control and accuracy.

Table 1 provides addresses for suppliers of bowling equipment.

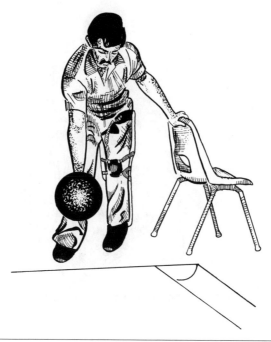

Figure 2.   Chairs are one of several devices that can be used by bowlers needing a little extra stability.

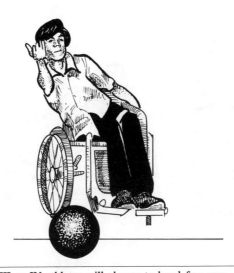

Figure 3.   Many Class III or IV athletes will choose to bowl free-arm.

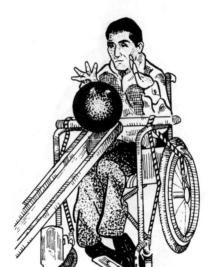

Figure 4.   Elastic rope is used to secure a wooden ramp to the bowler's wheelchair.

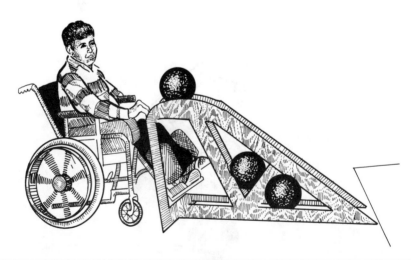

Figure 5.   Extra bowling balls are incorporated into the bowling ramp's design to provide stability.

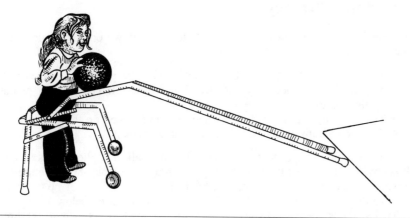

Figure 6.   Rubber tips and wheels protect the wooden floor. This ramp attaches directly to the athlete's walker.

Table 1   Bowling Equipment Suppliers

Philip Faas[a]
3226 Bayon Placido Blvd. N.E.
St. Petersburg, FL 33703
    813-526-5668

Recreation Unlimited, Inc.[b]
820 Woodend Road
Stratford, CT 06497
    203-384-0802

R & B Products[b]
1031 Navajo Trail So. Dr.
Indianapolis, IN 46260

Robert E. Lee[b]
Lee's Lanes
RFD #2
Mason City, IA 50401

George Snyder[c]
5809 NE 21st Avenue
Ft. Lauderdale, FL 33308
    305-772-6526

Apparel Unlimited[d]
6970 – 38th Street N.
Pinellas Park, FL 33565
    813-525-5109

Barker's Bowlium, Inc.[d]
2659 E. 75th Street
Chicago, IL 60649

BAN – North American Recreation[a b c d]
Box 7399
Dallas, TX 75209
    1-800-527-7415
    1-800-442-3451 (in Texas)

Flag House Inc.[a b d]
18 West 18th Street
New York, NY 10011
    212-989-9700

[a]Bowling sticks. [b]Ramps. [c]Ring ball holders. [d]Snap handle balls.

Coaching Strategy

The total number of pins a player is able to knock down on any single roll of the ball is a function of three variables:

- The accuracy with which the ball is delivered into the pocket (or, in the case of a spare shot, the accuracy with which it follows the best line for picking up the spare)
- The amount, if any, of the spin and/or curve placed on the ball
- The momentum of the ball (i.e., weight × velocity)

The momentum is dependent on the speed of the ball multiplied by its weight. It is obvious, then, that the heaviest regulation ball available should be used by a ramp bowler. Accuracy is controlled by the bowler's choice of ramp positions. (It also depends on curve and/or spin, but that is discussed below.)

Two methods are generally accepted for aiming the ball in bowling: (a) direct alignment, or simply pointing or aiming the ramp at the pins, and (b) spot bowling, or using the spots at the foul line and/or the arrows embedded in the lane surface to provide reference points for aiming the ball. The method chosen by any individual bowler depends on trial and error and the relative success encountered with a particular method; in other words, personal preference.

The amount of spin and/or curve placed on a ball as it leaves the ramp depends on the technique of the bowler's release (push) and the placement of the ball on the ramp. Plugged bowling balls can be modified so as to be heavier on one side than the other. This allows the bowler to align the ball on the ramp in a variety of ways so that a spin or curve will be added (see Figure 7).

The most important coaching advice that can be given to a bowler is to work toward consistency in every aspect of the approach to the game. Bowling is not a sport of brute strength or power, but of finesse.

Staffing Needs

In general, the following guidelines have been found to contribute to efficient (and therefore more enjoyable) bowling sessions:

- If manual scoring sheets are being used, assign two helpers to each lane of sedentary bowlers. One person keeps score and one retrieves the ball, positions it according to the bowler's instructions, and moves the ramp only as instructed. Make certain each bowler and his or her helper understand that helpers are *not* to make any suggestions as to ball placement, ramp position, or pins to aim for in picking up a spare. Failure by the bowler's assistant to adhere to the rules can result in the disqualification of the bowler.
- If automated scoring is used, one person can program several scoring machines and need not stay on a particular lane. In other words, only one person needs to be assigned to stay permanently on each lane.
- Sedentary bowlers should bowl an entire game with no interruption; ambulatory bowling team members can rotate after completing each frame.

Using the methods explained above, it has been our experience, based on several years of league bowling, that a team of five to seven bowlers using two lanes can bowl two complete games each in roughly two hours.

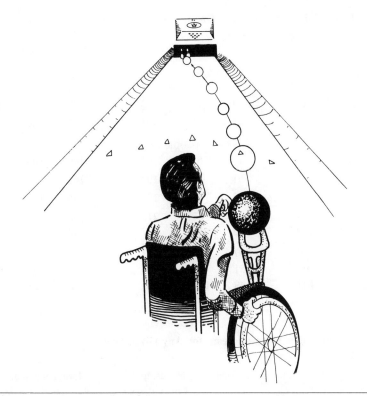

Figure 7. Modified plugged balls can help in aiming for the more difficult shots.

Handicapping Methods for Score Comparison

Below are some guidelines for establishing handicaps for competition. It should be stressed that only when handicapping procedures are applied consistently and without exception to every bowler in a league can handicapping be an accurate and fair method of comparing scores of different classifications of bowlers.

1. Consider a minimum of eight scratch games in computing a bowler's average. Obviously, the fewer games considered, the less representative the average will be.
2. Round the average to the nearest whole number of pins; subtract this number from 200 (if the average is 200 or more, no handicap is computed; the bowler is simply considered a scratch bowler). The average subtracted from 200 equals the individual's handicap. For example, a bowler who averaged 134 for eight games would have a handicap of 66 (200 − 134 = 66).
3. If possible, use the bowler's final eight games or bowling training sessions from his or her previous season of bowling to compute the average and handicap. In most cases, this method is far more representative of the bowler's abilities than the first games of a new season. It also encourages bowlers to bowl up to their potential early in the season (see Table 2).

Table 2   Determining Averages and Handicaps

Games		Team 1				Team 2	
	A	B	C	D	E	F	G
1	90	47	14	190	130	97	100
2	87	62	27	201	152	99	107
3	63	12	48	200	147	106	94
4	101	17	51	203	140	109	119
5	117	51	38	199	159	112	130
6	80	75	74	185	165	115	85
7	103	60	67	215	146	93	91
8	119	83	63	197	148	92	93
Total	760	407	382	1,600	1,187	823	817
Average	95	51	48	200	148	103	102
Handicap	105	149	152	0	52	97	98

Table 3   Determining a Winning Team for Any Given Day

Player	Game 1	Game 2	Total	Handicap × games played	Individual score total pins + handicap
Team 1					
A	96	101	197	105 × 2 = 210	197 + 210 = 407
B	47	33	80	149 × 2 = 298	80 + 149 = 229
C	32	87	119	152 × 2 = 304	119 + 152 = 271
D	195	207	402	0	402 + 0 = 402
Team 2					
E	121	137	258	52 × 2 = 104	258 + 104 = 362
F	83	106	189	97 × 2 = 194	189 + 194 = 383
G	98	117	215	98 × 2 = 196	215 + 196 = 411

Team totals[a]

Team 1[b]	Team 2
407	362
271	383
402	411
1,080	1,156

[a]Team 2 won by 76 points. [b]Player D was not included in the total due to the unequal numbers of players per team.

4. When comparing scores of two teams who have an unequal number of bowlers, drop the lowest scores of the team with the greater number of members. For example, if Team 1 has four bowlers and Team 2 has only three bowlers, disregard the scores of the lowest-scoring member of Team 1. This would leave three sets of scores to be compared to the three sets of scores of Team 2 (see Table 3).

Note

For more information, contact: American Wheelchair Bowling Association, Inc., N. 54 W. 15858 Lark Spur Lane, Menomonee, WI 53051, (414) 781-6876

References

Lane, J., & Schoof, D. *Wheelchair Bowling*. Huntington Beach, CA: Wheelchair Bowlers of Southern California.

Nunnenkamp, B. (1976, July). Bowling from a wheelchair. *Sports 'N Spokes*, pp. 17–19.

Wheelchair specialized equipment. (1975, September). *Sports 'N Spokes*, p. 2.

Cycling Techniques

Bob Accorsi
Pat Pride

Cycling has generally been considered a European sport. It is, however, becoming increasingly more popular in the U.S. due largely to the current fitness boom and the recent success of U.S. riders in international and Olympic competitions. This popularity has spilled over to CP sports, where both bicycle and tricycle events are offered within United States Cerebral Palsy Athletic Association's (USCPAA) competitive program.

A good bicyclist or tricyclist must combine athletic ability, extensive training, good quality properly fitting equipment, and smart riding. Here are a few suggestions on reaching your highest potential in these areas.

Equipment

Your equipment should be as lightweight as possible and well maintained and lubricated. If you cannot afford an entire new bicycle or tricycle we suggest you try to invest in lightweight wheels with good hubs and high pressure tires. When selecting new tires for tricycles, be sure not to select tires too large for the frame. Instability will occur if you do.

The bicycle's fit is very important to provide comfortable and efficient pedaling. The size of your frame should allow you to straddle your bike in front of the saddle with both feet flat on the ground, and still have 1-in. clearance between your groin and the bicycle's top tube.

When selecting a tricycle, coaches must take into account comfort and the athlete's height and arm length. The athlete should be slightly bent over while in the seated position, with both hands on the handlebars. This slightly bent technique reduces "air drag" by making the rider a little more aerodynamic. The frame must be conducive to this position while maintaining comfort and efficiency (see Figure 1).

Next to the frame, saddle (seat) height is tremendously important. Most people ride with their seat too high. To test saddle height, put your heels on the pedals and back pedal. If your heels do not reach the pedals during the full rotation, lower your seat. If your legs are two different lengths, we suggest that you compromise the height between both legs. The athlete's legs should be slightly bent with the heel in the down position on the pedal at the bottom of the rotation. The saddle position may initially feel cramped, but it provides better positioning for a snap in your legs.

In addition, bike shoes and toe clips are essential to assist the athlete in the proper pedaling technique. The combination of both will provide the stability to

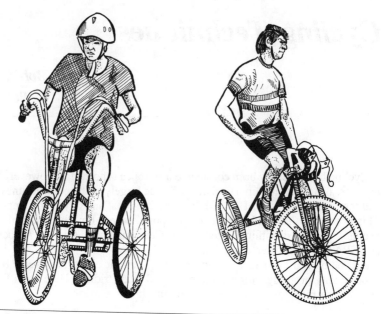

Figure 1.   Sport tricycles allow a great many athletes to participate in cycling who because of balance difficulties are unable to ride a two-wheeled bike.

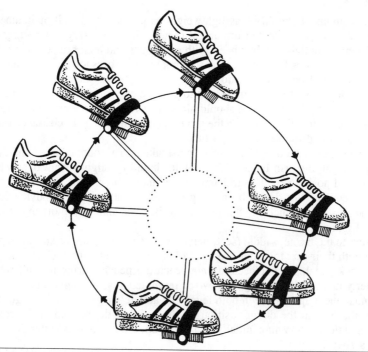

Figure 2.   The pedaling motion.

hold the feet in place and to allow the athlete the full pedal stroke. And, finally, athletes are required to wear some type of safety helmet during competition. Coaches and athletes should consult bicycle dealers for the best fitting and safest helmet available.

Pedaling Techniques

Many people think that pedaling high gears is the best exercise and training, but too much pushing of big gears may often result in knee strain and injuries. You'll ride faster and longer and get a great workout if you spin lower gears, and spin them fast. Ride in a gear that is low enough that you notice only slight effort on the pedals. Ride these gears in a quick cadence (pedaling speed) of about 70 revolutions per minute. A quick cadence is your ticket to fast riding and also better cardiovascular conditioning. Your legs will get stronger, fatigue less, and move faster.

Remember to pedal in a circle with the ball of your foot over the pedal (Figure 2). Try to train with toe clips and straps that secure your feet to the pedal. In this way, your pedaling effort can pull on the pedals during the full rotation. Feel your feet and effort going around—not up and down.

Training

During your preseason training, you should work on putting in many miles of training, spinning low gears. Work on riding long distances to build up your lungs and heart. As you get closer to competition, emphasis will turn to interval training. Because USCPAA cycling events include 1,500-, 3,000-, 5,000-, and 10,000-m time trials, which are relatively short distances for bicycle races, athletes must be able to maintain high speeds during the entire race. Interval training is excellent for developing speed.

Although very important, we suggest that riders do interval training only twice each week. Too much interval training taxes the body and can cause sport-related injuries. Also, coaches should never plan interval training 2 days in a row.

The principle of interval workouts is simple: The athlete rides hard for short work intervals and is allowed to rest between each work interval. During the work intervals, riders maintain a level of effort that would tire them out if they were not given a chance to recover during the rest interval. The high level of effort taxes leg muscles and the cardiovascular system so they get stronger. Interval training is the fastest way to build up aerobic fitness. During interval training, a rider must spin higher gears than usual at a faster cadence than they normally ride.

Athletes should never get on their bike or trike cold. Always warm up properly, utilizing leg and upper body stretching techniques including knee bends, arm and head circles, hip and trunk rotations, leg raises, and calf stretches (whenever possible).

Also, before starting interval workout, riders should ride steadily for at least 20 min to warm up. Now comes the hard part. Set the bike in a higher gear than the athlete would normally ride, and spin that gear at 90 revolutions per minute or more. Try to begin your interval training with this schedule:

- Two 2-minute intervals—which means 2 minutes of spinning a high gear, very fast.
- Two 1-minute intervals
- Two 1/2-minute intervals

As the rider begins to feel more conditioned for interval training, attempt to do several 3- and 4-minute intervals. These will be your key to victory.

Time Trials

A good start is very important in the short distance time trials that are held in USCPAA competition. The riders should practice their start with their coach as much as possible. Have the coach hold the back of the seat while you stand up on the foot pedals. He or she may steady the bike or trike by placing his or her legs on either side of the wheel(s). The pedal of the strongest leg should be positioned at 1 or 2 o'clock. The athlete's weight should be as far forward as possible while still being comfortable.

Just prior to the start, the rider should breathe deeply several times to get as much oxygen as possible. Teach your riders to put some pressure on the pedals so that when the command comes, they can get off quickly. Have them start out of the saddle, and stay out of the saddle until they have those pedals really buzzing. Riders should feel like they are running on their bicycle or tricycle. Bikes may sway from side to side from the intensity of their effort, but don't worry about that unless they have poor balance. Swaying may be more dangerous for trike riders where balance is definitely a factor. Often coaches will have to teach trike riders to find a happy medium between balance and pedaling power.

If your rider feels very uncomfortable and unbalanced in a standing position, he or she may have to start in a seated position. This will be less productive and slower at the start. The standing start feels unbalanced initially, even for able-bodied riders, so attempt it several times before disregarding it.

Racing the Distance

After getting a good fast start, the tendency is for the rider to sit down too soon. If their balance is good, they should stay up running on those pedals a little longer. When they do sit down, they should pedal it up to almost a sprint, but hold back from a complete burst because they still have a distance to go. The rest is not going to be easy—it is painful. The rider is racing against the clock, and he or she can't let up because the clock keeps ticking.

One mistake cyclists make in these short races is to try to save energy in the beginning and not make a good start. Riders have to make every second count because they can never be regained.

Two important things for coaches to remember are, first, have your riders go to the starting line warmed up completely. If they are not warmed up, their muscles and hearts cannot work to full capacity. Second, have them ride as straight a line as possible.

Finally, in USCPAA, the riders will start 1 minute apart, with start and finish times recorded and used to find the best overall time for the distance. The man ahead of your rider is called his minute man, and it does provide some incentive to try to catch him. Coaches should have athletes thinking about the minute man, but not concentrating solely on catching him. Remind your riders that they have a complete race to ride.

Training Card

Athletes should be encouraged to keep a daily record of their training. This helps coaches and riders identify progress, problems, and attitudes toward training. Here is some suggested information to put on your daily training card:

1. Day and date
2. Pulse—Count beats for 15 seconds, multiply by 4.
3. Weight (in pounds)
4. Description of training ride
   - Distance—Record miles covered.
   - Time—Record the amount of time taken to cover this distance.
   - Gearing—Note the number of teeth on the front chain ring and the number on the back sprocket.
   - Type of course—Record whether it is hilly, flat, and so forth.
5. Interval training—List the amount and length of your interval training. For example, if you have done three 2-minute intervals, record it as 3 × 2 minutes.
6. Other training—Record any and all types of athletic training you have done that day.

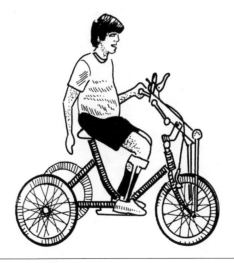

Figure 3. Arm-driven tricycle.

Cycling Alternatives

As in many sports, cycling can be and is often a very successful recreational activity. The introduction of tricycles and adaptive equipment has allowed many athletes to participate in competitive and recreational riding who otherwise would not be able to participate.

One type of tricycle gaining in popularity is the arm-driven cycle shown in Figure 3. Arm-driven tricycles are available commercially and offer a great deal of independence to paraplegic riders.

Conclusion

USCPAA cycling is still within developmental stages. Continued research into low-cost, custom-built equipment, training techniques, and increased competitive opportunities will help foster a new trend in cycling for disabled athletes.

For more information, contact United States Cycling Federation, 1750 E. Boulder Street, Colorado Springs, CO 80909, 303-578-4581; or, Bob Accorsi, USCPAA Cycling Technical Advisor, 228 Florence Road, Florence, MA 01060.

Note

For more information, contact United States Cycling Federation, 1750 E. Boulder Street, Colorado Springs, CO 80909, 303-578-4581; or, Bob Accorsi, USCPAA Cycling Technical Advisor, Recreation and Leisure Services, Springfield College, Springfield, MA 01109.

Reference

Simes, J. (1976). *Winning bicycle racing*. Chicago: Contemporary Books.

Soccer Strategies for the Beginning Coach and Team

Paul Roper
Phil Roberts

Soccer is, many would agree, a game requiring great skill. It demands finesse, strength, endurance, speed, ball skill, and strategy. During a game a player will require several of these components at any one time. How, then, is the beginning coach to organize and prepare individuals for team play?

An initial concern must be to gain some understanding of the principal components required of the sport.[1] The coach of a team organized to compete under United States Cerebral Palsy Athletic Association (USCPAA) rules must assess demands according to the number of players, the class representation of these players, and the size of the playing field. All too often the coach becomes overly concerned with tight ball control on the mistaken assumption that this is what the game is all about. Realistically, this does not constitute the most important concern for beginning teams.

This chapter attempts to put forward the following four basic assumptions:

1. There are certain key areas of the field.
2. Players must be able to kick and pass the ball accurately for a reasonable distance.
3. Soccer is a dynamic, not a static game.
4. Coaches will have the ability to effectively evaluate each athlete's playing ability.

Having a clear understanding of these concepts will greatly enhance a coach's ability to organize a cerebral palsy (CP) soccer team.

USCPAA Rule Adaptations

Although the game is played primarily under Federation Internationale de Football Association (FIFA) rules, there are a few changes incorporated to make the game more competitive for CP athletes. This article will begin by briefly discussing two: the number of players (and representation of certain classes), and the size of the field. Specifics on the remaining changes can be found in a current USCPAA rule book.

In accordance with USCPAA rules, a team of *seven* players (not 11 as in able-bodied soccer) must play at least one Class V or Class VI athlete and no more than four Class VIII athletes at any given time. There will exist a wide variety of ambulation ability among athletes in these four classes. Due to their more involved lower body, it may be to your advantage to play your Class V and VI athletes in a defensive position, or they may be your best choice for goal keeper. Your Class VIII athletes will usually provide the manpower for your offensive front line. You should, however, look at the strengths and weaknesses of all your players and determine how they each fit the requirements of the different positions and different game situations. As always, the key is to know your athletes. There will be Class VI athletes that are very capable of playing a wing or inside forward position, as well as Class VIII athletes who were unable to meet those same demands.

The second change in able-bodied rules in the reduction of the field size from a length and width of at least 100 and 64 m to a 80- by 60-m field. The combination of a smaller field and fewer players can be very deceptive. In fact, there is still a large amount of space to be covered by seven players.

When players are given large expanses in which to move, they will invariably be tempted to chase all over the field. This is exactly what the coach does not want his or her side to do. Those who run around excessively soon become fatigued with a subsequent loss of skill and interest. While the coach would wish this for the opposition, a concern for his or her team must be to conserve energy through efficient work output. Our first two assumptions that should be considered in this type of situation are (a) there are certain key areas of the field and (b) players must be able to kick and pass the ball accurately for a reasonable distance.

Key Areas of the Field

In soccer, the area in front of the goal (penalty area) is a key section of the field. Accordingly, there should always be a player to defend this area, and only under extreme circumstances should this player be drawn away from that position. This player represents the last line of defense and is sometimes referred to as the *sweeper*. Likewise, an attacking player should be near or ready to enter this section at the opponent's end of the field. Figure 1a shows this key area for defense.

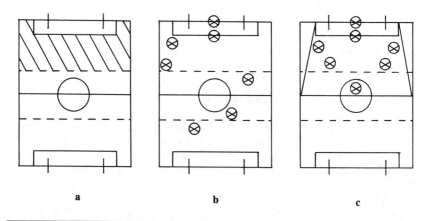

a   b   c

Figure 1.   (a) Key area for defense, (b) offensive distribution of players, and (c) defensive distribution of players.

It can be seen that this area may be extended forward up to a third of the entire field. This is the *defensive third*. Players should be distributed out from this area in positions that are dependent upon ball possession (offense), or possession by the opposition (defense). If on offense, midfield forwards must spread to maximize distances from the opposition and from each other in order to use as much of the playing field as possible (Figure 1b). When on defense, players should collapse back in a funnel-like fashion to the key areas (Figure 1c). Viewing the field in thirds will also assist in planning for offense or defensive positioning. The middle third of the field is a link between offense and defense. Few teams will be capable of kicking the ball over this area and it is from there that your offense or defense must ideally begin.

Working the Ball

The other aspect, the player's ability to kick and pass the ball accurately for a reasonable distance, is important so he or she can "work" the ball around the field and use their individual efforts effectively. When a team is on offense, moving the ball wide to the side and encouraging defenders to chase out will tire the opposition at the same time, causing them to vacate that middle key section.

Just as with basketball, the idea in soccer is to advance the ball into the opposition's area of the field and to open up access to a scoring position. Also, as in basketball, this may require a circuitous route or a direct route, dependent upon the opposition's defense posture. Often, there is a need to draw defensive players out of the key area and to coincide your player's movement into that space with the arrival of the ball. In this way, scoring opportunities are created such that most goals are scored from within the penalty area.

When a player gains possession of the ball, he or she must gain composure and space in which to work. A player should then ask the following questions:

1. Can I score?
2. Can another player score if I pass the ball to him or her?
3. Is anyone in a better position than myself to advance the ball forward without loss of possession?

If the answer to each of the above is "no," then that player must advance the ball by dribbling or hold the ball until another team member comes to assist. The worse thing a player can do is to kick the ball into his or her own key area, or to an area where the opposition has the possibility of gaining possession. In a difficult or potentially dangerous situation, the motto should be, "if in doubt, kick it out"; this gives your team time to regroup.

Looking at Defense

Players who do not have the ball should either (a) get into position to receive a pass or, (b) position themselves to defend should possession be lost. One cardinal rule is that a defensive player in such a position should always have a position between the ball and their own goal.

If the opposition has ball possession, then the player nearest the ball must delay the advance of the ball while his or her teammates regain defensive positions. Defensive positioning may be either soft zone, where each person covers an area of the field, or man-to-man, where a player stays with a particular member of the opposition. The choice of which defense to use will depend on a number of factors: skill level of your team versus your opponent, fatigue, and the score. When defending, the cardinal rule given above should include the added condition that the defender must be between the persons he or she is marking and the goal. In this way, the defender keeps the opposition and the ball in front in order to watch both. A defender should never overcommit (i.e., make a desperate tackle) in a situation where the opposition has a chance to score. Rather, he or she should wait for the person with the ball to make a wrong move or mistake. This is called containing. This is unlike an offensive player who, when taking a defensive role, should hustle the opposition to force an error. A final suggestion for defensive players is that they should not chase the ball around the field; rather, they should stay within a particular area (zone) or with a particular player of the opposite team.

Dynamic Skills

Our third basic assumption is that soccer is a dynamic, open, and fluid game. Passing, kicking accurately, and gaining control of the ball are the most important skills. All too often coaches think that close ball control, that is, dribbling, feinting, turning, thigh traps, and so on are the first skills to learn. Typically, training consists of players doing drills that are static in nature and bear little resemblance to game play. Only infrequently do situations arise in a game that are static in nature. A majority of the time the ball and the player are moving; other times the ball or the player is moving, and rarely are both set. Those situations where it does occur are described as set plays, as in goal kicks and corner kicks. Therefore, players should be encouraged to practice while either they or the ball are in motion.

Stationary drills should be made dynamic as soon as players have sufficient proficiency. For example, players are encouraged to change from kicking a stationary ball to kicking a ball that is rolled to them. They should then progress

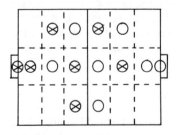

Figure 2. Field divided into designated playing areas and occupied by opposing players in order to encourage passing.

to kicking a ball while they are moving and finally, as they dribble a ball forward. Such practices should later progress by involving passive and then active opposition.

When transferring these skills into a lead up game, it might be wise to have players remain within a designated space on the field. The field can be marked into grids in which a player must stand. Alternate opposing players so that to advance the ball to a scoring position, a team must pass accurately past someone from the opposing team (Figure 2).

When the coach decides to use less structured formats, emphasis should still be on the need to stay in particular zones and for individuals to be fully aware of key areas on the field. Training should begin to involve dribbling over distances of up to 12 m. The next consideration for the coach once these concepts have been introduced is what to do when certain set plays are needed.

Player Assessment

Our final assumption involves the coach's ability to accurately assess an athlete's playing ability. Several secondary considerations may affect an athlete's ability to play soccer competitively.

Fitness

Of all the ambulatory events offered by USCPAA, soccer may be the most demanding. Good track athletes may not always make good soccer players. The fact that they have been trained for the 100 m dash does not mean they will be able to handle 40 minutes of continual running. Unless properly trained, lack of endurance may be the hidden disability of a number of your players.

Past Playing Experience

A number of your players may not acquire the necessary skills as easily as others because they have never had the opportunity to play the game. They may have, for any number of reasons, been excluded from physical education classes as well as participation in community-based soccer leagues. Your players may have developmental delays in kicking skills and difficulty understanding basic offensive and defensive strategies. You may find yourself teaching a teenager basic kicking skills often already mastered by a nine- or ten-year-old. Again, skill acquisition may be slow with some athletes, so be patient.

Sight

Do not automatically blame poor kicking and dribbling skills on a player's clumsiness. Your athlete may have some type of visual/perception problems that will limit their eye-foot coordination (an obvious skill necessary to the game). Players with vision or perception difficulties may be more effective playing a defensive position. With training for a specific position, a player may be able to more than adequately compensate for a vision or perceptual problem.

Hearing

Deafness may not directly affect an athlete's individual playing ability; however, it becomes very important in a team sport. Communication is vital! Coaches will find it necessary to establish some type of system that will enable players to communicate with a hearing-impaired athlete throughout the game.

Balance

Obviously, balance and foot coordination are primary factors to be considered in ambulatory soccer. The degree to which an athlete's gait is involved, limiting movement and stability, may dictate which position they can hope to play. Some positions require much more running, agility, and ball control than others, making them unlikely positions for players with extreme gait involvements, regardless of the level of enthusiasm.

Conclusion

A clear understanding of the four concepts outlined within this chapter should provide a coach with an adequate starting point for the beginning of a soccer team.

Soccer provides a rare opportunity for Class V, VI, VII, and VIII athletes to play a team sport equitably. The benefits of such an activity are too numerous to list. Don't take our word for it start a team and see for yourself.

Note

For more information regarding current national and international, youth and senior league able-bodied soccer, contact: United States Soccer Federation, United States Olympic Training Center, 1750 Boulder Street, Colorado Springs, CO 80909-5791, (303) 632-5551 or (303) 578-4678

References

Bauer, G. (1982). *How to succeed at soccer*. NY: Sterling Publishing.

McGettigan, J.P. (1980). *Complete book of drills for winning soccer*. West Nyack, NY: Parker.

Vogelsinger, H. (1970). *Winning soccer skills and techniques*. West Nyack, NY: Parker.

Wade, A. (1978). *Coach yourself soccer*. Dewsbury, West Yorks, Great Britain: E.P. Publishers.

Wheelchair Team Handball

Dave Stephenson
Mike Mushett

Wheelchair team handball, formerly known as wheelchair soccer, is an exciting game that combines rules and strategies of soccer, basketball, hockey, and team handball. Since its inclusion in the 1979 National Cerebral Palsy Games, wheelchair handball has grown in popularity for two basic reasons. First, it is the first game designed for all classes of athletes with cerebral palsy (CP), giving each class an equal role in the game. Second, the game provides an overall learning experience and opportunity for personal growth unmatched by any other event.[1] In 1986, the international governing body, Cerebral Palsy–International Sports and Recreation Association (CP-ISRA), changed its name from wheelchair soccer to wheelchair team handball because it was the consensus of the Sports Technical Committee that the rules tended to be more similar to team handball than soccer.

Facility and Equipment

Coaches should refer to the United States Cerebral Palsy Athletic Association (USCPAA) Rules Manual for specific dimensions and requirements. In summary, a typical basketball court, indoors or out, is satisfactory. An indoor court is preferred to an outdoor court because wood is a safer surface to play and fall on. A 10-in. playground ball and two soccer goals meeting the rule book dimensions are needed to get started.

As the skill level improves and level of competition becomes more serious, the team may need to purchase specially designed sports wheelchairs for the more mobile players. You may find your players buying their own chairs as they provide a greater degree of daily independence as well as increased court ability. One last note on equipment: The game is very hard on chairs, that is, spokes and bolts, so it is important to have spare parts and tools to make on-the-spot repairs. Spoke guards and antitip devices are also suggested. Coaches should refer to the section of this manual pertaining to wheelchair selection for more details.

Players by Positions

The team will consist of nine players: two goalies, two defensive players in front of the goalies, and five offensive players. Although this formation is used by many teams, it depends on the individual coaching strategies in specific game situations and on types of players available. For example, four offensive players and three defensive players is common, and in certain game situations (your team is behind) seven offensive players can and have been used.

The rule book presently requires four players on the court from Classes I, II, III, and VI-quad (an ambulatory Class VI who is quadraplegic); one from each class allowing for substitution down but not up. For example, you could have four Class I athletes playing, but not four Class III athletes. The remaining five players can be any combination of athletes from Classes IV, V, and VI (non-quadraplegic). This rule must be kept in mind when developing your team roster.

The *offensive line* usually consists of Class IV and V players who possess better ball control. However, there may be a role for a strong Class III who can block and catch and possibly a role for a Class I who has above average mobility and is able to block for the ball handlers.

The *defensive line* in front of the goal must be able to break up the opponents' offensive patterns, keep opponents off the crease, and block shots. This requires good range of motion in the shoulders, a good degree of mobility, and the ability to work closely with his or her fellow defenseperson, thus creating teamwork.

The two goalies must be mobile to be able to turn to face the attack, have a good range of motion with the ability to catch, and be able to work as a team. This position is the most important and often the most difficult. The goalies can't be afraid of contact such as being hit in the face. They must be alert even if the ball is not close by and have the sense for the goal's vulnerable areas.

There is room in this game for everyone. The trick is evaluating abilities, teaching appropriate skills, and molding everyone's talents into a team (see Figure 1). It does not take a lot of Class IV and V athletes to make a championship team. The starting offensive line-up for the 1985 national championship team, the Houston Challengers, only had one Class IV. The remaining front line were from Classes I, II, III, or VI-quad.

Evaluating Ability

A coach needs to take the time to evaluate each player's ability level. Ask yourself, are they unable to catch, dribble, or pass because they don't have the ability

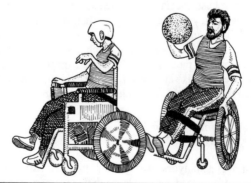

Figure 1.   A Class I athlete in a power wheelchair can often provide good blocking for a team's ball handlers.

or because they have never been taught? When did they begin to participate in organized sports? Do you have teenagers or adults who have never had "little league sports" experiences? If so, you need to teach these skills from the beginning.

Check for visual problems that may be making the skills more difficult to perform. Perceptual difficulties may be compensated for with proper training techniques. The eyes are the key to almost every skill. Do they watch the ball into their hands? If not, can they if given a verbal command to keep their eyes on the ball? If they can't watch the ball or learn to watch, then perceptual problems need to be overcome. You will need to investigate specific techniques to overcome these problems.

A coach will need to determine each player's learning ability. Players will fall into one of three levels: the ability to perform a certain skill successfully; the ability to learn how to achieve a skill; and the inability to ever learn that skill. In the first two levels there will be, of course, various levels of accomplishments, depending on the individual, with improvement usually needed in some way. As a coach it is imperative that skill abilities be matched with positions. Players should know what they need to practice in order to improve for their specific positions. This, of course, will match what they will be asked to do in a game situation. Teammates should know who can catch a pass and who cannot, who can dribble and who cannot. Each player's job description will center around *all* of his or her abilities. For example, during an in-bounds play, the player putting the ball into play must be a player who can pass the ball correctly and consistently. He or she passes to the player who can catch while moving. A "safety value" player will be nearby who is able to catch while being stationary and who can also make an immediate return pass to someone else. Molding your player's abilities into team play is the key to a successful team.

Fundamental Skills

There are four fundamental skills to wheelchair handball; passing, dribbling, catching, and wheelchair mobility (such as pivoting, stopping, cutting, faking, and moving backward). The more advanced skills of passing, dribbling, and catching while moving, moving with the ball in the lap, blocking, and executing the "pic 'n roll" and the "give 'n go" cannot be successfully introduced until the fundamental skills are acquired.

Teaching and reinforcing fundamental skills should be tailored to the ability level of the athletes. This is easier said than done considering the wide range of abilities you may have on your team. For beginners, start with stationary drills with players close together. Then gradually increase the distance. Group players by ability level, thus enabling you to run more difficult drills with higher skilled players, while at the same time running easier drills with other players. Although you should not allow drills to dominate your practice time, it is appropriate to devote the first two or three practice sessions entirely to drills and conditioning in order to develop a solid foundation before moving on to scrimmages. During these practices, you can do the evaluation of skill levels that were discussed above. It will also give the newcomers a chance to get a feel for the game and the other players. As soon as your players are proficient with stationary drills, include motion. Very few things are done in wheelchair team handball in a stationary position.

Passing

Players need to learn all forms of passing; the out-of-bounds pass, the chest pass, the baseball pass, the bounce pass, and even passing with the foot and/or wheelchair. Of course, passing also implies catching. Both can be taught in the same drills. Position your coaching staff to work with each group. Take the time to instruct those who can learn how to pass and catch using the proper method. How do you catch a bounce pass? How do you catch a pass that is on the side of the wheelchair without falling out? Give them the motor tools to work with and then allow your players to mold the skills into their individual ability levels. Players need to practice passing and catching with and without a bounce, short and long distances, and from stationary and moving positions or at targets. The coach needs to learn a player's passing distance. Are they a short passer or a long passer? What kind of pass can they catch? What kind of pass can they make? Who is consistent and who cannot be consistent?

Shots on goal are similar to passing with some finer techniques added. Of course, the drills will be different than passing ones. You will need to set the drills up with goalies and defensepersons to block shots. The types of shots will be similar to passes, except the object is that they should not be able to be caught. This leads to introducing players to the vulnerable areas of the goal (Figure 2). They include the high corners, the middle, and the low corners of the goal. Good goalies can read where the ball is going, anticipating their moves before the shot is made.

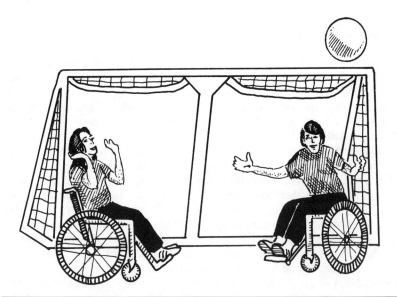

Figure 2.   Coaches must teach goalies to defend the vulnerable areas of the goal.

Consequently, the most successful shots are those that catch the goalies out of position. Coaches need to teach certain tricks including eye fakes, quick passes to the weak side when the goalies have shifted to face a strong side shot, and the bounce shot that makes the goalie bend down to catch a ball that is now bouncing over their head. Coaches, of course, need to teach your goalies not to be taken in by the fakes.

Following up shots for possible rebounds should always be taught in conjunction with shots on goal. Most goals seem to be scored with the goalies out of position after a rebounded shot is caught and reshot. Rebound shots tend to be more successful than the initial shot simply because the goalies do not have the time to react.

Dribbling

In many cases, dribbling can be a very difficult skill. However, in order for your team to be successful, each player will need to learn how to dribble in some fashion. Successful dribbling will depend on a player's functional ability and can include dribbling and passing with the foot or wheelchair, a single bounce in a stationary position, or dribbling while moving. Coaches should teach players with the higher skill levels to dribble without looking at the ball and while on the move (see Figure 3).

Dribbling is a skill easily practiced at home. If possible, your program should provide balls to those players needing extra practice at home.

Teams should always work drills and scrimmages with the 3-second rule in effect. Coach the players that they have a choice on where to get rid of the ball. If they cannot pass to a teammate, tell them to take a shot on the goal, dribble it on the floor, or off of an opponent's wheelchair out-of-bounds within the allotted 3 seconds. The players can always toss, throw, or kick the ball toward the opponent's goal. This is called a *clearing-out pass*. If it simply goes out-of-bounds on their end of the court, then it is an excellent defensive move. Your team then can regroup in the offense court, playing hard defense while hoping for a turnover close to the goal.

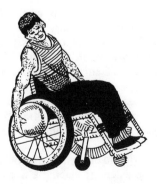

Figure 3. Advanced skills include teaching athletes to use the wheelchair's rotating wheel to recover a loose ball off the floor.

Evaluating and teaching skills is an ongoing process. Coaches need to be patient and positive. Accentuate the individual abilities by designing game strategies around these abilities. Not everyone will be able to learn textbook skills, but each of their skill levels needs to be enhanced to the optimal level. More importantly, all of their abilities need to be molded into the team strategy and into the execution of their positions. By focusing on everyone's abilities, you will give each player the feeling that they can do something positive for the team. Each player will have a role and a specific responsibility.

Teamwork

The ability of a team to successfully coordinate its players and their abilities in a given situation is teamwork. Players must learn when to pass and when not to pass and when to shoot and when not to shoot. The learning of what to do and when to do it is all a part of educating your players to the strategies of the game. Essential to teaching teamwork is understanding that everyone has a role and that it is only when everyone is doing his or her job (including the coaches) that the team will be most successful. Scoring goals means nothing if your goalies are allowing the opponent to score twice as many. The players on the bench must have an ongoing awareness of the game. Without it they will be lost upon entering the game. The goalies must work together, the fullbacks must work together, and the wings and center(s) must work together with the blockers.

Teamwork is cooperation among all of the team, from an immediate and smooth transition from offense to defense to the wing positioning him- or herself to receive a rebound or back door pass from the center, to a player on the bench lending his wheelchair to the center when his wheelchair breaks irreparably. In order to achieve teamwork, each player must know his or her abilities and his or her job responsibilities. Teamwork is the name of the game.

Playbook

One way to make this learning process a little easier is through the use of a playbook. It will give the players an opportunity to learn away from practice as a supplement to the hands-on learning of practice sessions. A playbook should explain terminology of skills, key areas of the court, job responsibilities by position, game strategies, and general team expectations such as attendance and team rules.

The playbook will enable you to outline drills and plays as well as explain concepts of teamwork and offensive and defensive strategies. The playbook, if done right, will enable the players to speak the same language and enable you to talk with understanding.

The issuing of a playbook should carry a degree of responsibility, reinforcing the team concept even to the extent of placing a fine on the athlete if the book is lost. Make sure that you provide assistance in studying to those who have learning disabilities. This can be accomplished by contacting the parents to gain their help or having another coach provide tutoring.

Some tips in preparing your playbook follow. The terminology that you use is very important. What is a "high-post" or "back door" or a "crease?" Where is the outside lane or center lane? What is a fastbreak or a transition? Define specific areas of the court such as the deep court, center lane, and outside lane. This terminology will better enable you to define job descriptions.

Practice Sessions

It is important to develop, as soon as possible, a team structure, including a head coach, offensive and defensive coaches, assistant coaches, and captains. This will give coaches specific rules, key players the responsibilities of captains, and the head coach a way to delegate overall responsibilities.

Each practice should begin the same way with everyone having his or her own job. Players should be taught to be responsible for their own needs, including equipment, strapping, and warm-ups. Those athletes requiring assistance need to know how they can be helped because on a given day or season, a different coach may be responsible for attending to their needs. Coaches' jobs include strapping, making repairs, pumping tires, setting up goals, and assisting with warm-ups. An established routine before each practice will pay dividends all season long.

The practice season should flow in three stages. The first two or three practice sessions should focus on drills and conditioning, with the playbook given out at the first practice. These first sessions will give everyone time to learn what is expected. The second two or three sessions (maybe four) should be spent on half-court scrimmages for the purpose of instructing on plays, roles, positions, rules, and so on. The third stage, consisting of a majority of the sessions, should be spent on full-court scrimmages using a referee.

Drills

During drills is the time for athletes to practice and learn while the coaches evaluate skill levels. It is important that athletes are able to distinguish what they can and cannot do and at what level they can do it. This identification sets expectations in a proper perspective. Conditioning drills are important and have a place throughout the entire season. Coaches should not forget to evaluate speed in these drills as well as overall range of speed.

Half-Court Scrimmages

Half-court scrimmages are the next logical step, allowing you to add new aspects of the game in a progressive manner. This portion of the season enables a coach to control the pace of practice by stopping play when there is the need to instruct, substitute, and/or discuss new plays. Half-court play also allows defensive and offensive coaches the opportunities to work closely with their players. This is the time for setting expectations of players by position, areas of the court, and individual skill levels, as well as teaching your players the many options and choices they have in various game situations. Half-court sessions should progress from the offensive unit trying to score against just the goalies, to adding the defensive unit, to the five offensive players trying to score on nine defensive players.

The step between half-court and full-court scrimmages begins with teaching your players about starting the fastbreak; the transition game from how to start your offense and how to stop the opponent from starting their offensive. Full-court scrimmages should then begin with at least one coach acting as a referee. Although officiating is added at this point to reinforce the rules of three seconds, ramming, and so forth, it should not control the tempo of the scrimmage. Learning to play at game tempo is essential to the individual player's mental transition of thinking about what he or she is supposed to do and automatically doing it. Everything leading up to a full-court scrimmage is done in progression, setting the stage for this transition from a thinking response to an automatic response. This may be very difficult for some, so give it time.

Full-Court Scrimmages

It is during full-court scrimmages that players develop court sense, the ongoing awareness of the game situation. This involves knowing who is on offense and who is on defense, what their own job is, where they are on the court, and where their person is. Simple verbal clues from the bench or from key players on the floor should be used to remind everyone of their roles during a given situation. Communication, court balance, and team ball control will be several results of a series of well run full-court scrimmages.

"Practice makes perfect" implies that the more full-court scrimmages a team can have, the better. However, because of a number of reasons (lack of transportation is the single largest), many teams are unable to get enough players together often enough to hold complete full-court scrimmages. If your team is faced with this situation, there may be several solutions. For those players who do not have transportation problems, teams should first require both attendance and being on time and keep records. Second, never guarantee anyone a place on the team roster even if you have less than 15 players. You should have team rules, such as attendance, that must be met in order to be eligible to be selected to the team. After that, selection should be based on performance by class and position.

For those with transportation difficulties, coaches should attempt to develop some type of car pool within the team. And remember, a full-court scrimmage can be effectively done with any number of players. Seven on seven and six on six is fine as long as you keep the teams balanced by abilities. Always try to scrimmage the first string offensive unit and the second string defensive unit against the second string offensive unit and the first string defensive unit. You can also add coaches to the line-up to balance the sides out.

As a third solution, a number of teams across the country have addressed the problem of scrimmage time by turning to able-bodied clubs and organizations for competitive opportunities. Besides providing good program awareness, potential volunteer sources, great fund-raising opportunities, and an excellent chance for your players to meet people and make new friends, playing able-bodied groups has allowed several teams to expand their competitive schedules far beyond competition with other CP teams.

Although playing against able-bodied opponents can solve your problem of lack of competition, it also presents a few problems of its own. The first and most significant is number of wheelchairs. Most able-bodied individuals do not own their own wheelchairs, making it necessary for your program to come up with 8 to 10 extra wheelchairs in order to play. This may or may not be a concern. Some programs keep an inventory of used wheelchairs for various reasons. If your program does not, you should contact a local medical supply company or health organization. Explain the purpose of your program, and your need for 8 to 10 wheelchairs for 2 hours at a time. Offer to pick the wheelchairs up and return them, and your chances are very good that they will help you out.

Your second concern will be equality of play. It is our experience that most able-bodied groups that agree to play will have several individuals with fairly good athletic ability. Usually this ability is good enough to dominate ball possession. Although wheelchair mobility will be awkward and, depending on the strength of your defense, scoring goals may be very difficult, time of possession by means of passing and dribbling by your able-bodied opponents can be extensive. In order to counterbalance the obvious physical advantage, some CP teams have used two rule changes or "equalizers" in respect to able-bodied players. They include (a) *one-handed rule* that says once the player has obtained possession, any other manipulation of the ball (i.e., passing, dribbling, and shooting) must be done with one hand; if at any time after the player has initially gained possession, the second hand is used, the ball is turned over to the CP team and (b) *one goalie*. It is highly recommended, in order to ensure a realistic offensive threat on the part of the CP team, that the able-bodied team be limited to one goalie for a total of eight players versus two goalies and nine players of the CP team.

Conclusion

In closing, we suggest learning from experience. Start a team. Grow as a coach while your players grow as a team. Visit the nearest team to you. Observe. Ask questions. Play the game. Learn by doing. In most cases, starting a team will not be an easy task.

Finding enough players may be difficult at first. Once you begin, coaches and players should never stop looking for additional players. Recruitment is important to the continued success of any team.

Because the abilities of your athletes will be so varied, it will be your job to blend a wide range of abilities into one functional, well-skilled unit. Keep your expectations in perspective. When you do, wheelchair team handball provides the type of competitiveness, enjoyment, and independence that is both very real and beneficial for all those involved.

Note

For more information, sample playbooks and excellent videotapes on wheelchair team handball, contact: David Stephenson, Greater Houston Athletic Association, for the Physically Disabled, 1101 Post Oak Road, Suite 9-486, Houston, TX 77056, (713) 664-9007; or Mike Mushett, Michigan CP/LA Sports Association, P. O. Box 231, Garden City, MI 48135

Part IV

Considerations for the Future

Youth Sports:
Our Program's Future

Jeffery A. Jones

The extent of involvement of younger athletes in organized sports programs for the physically disabled has increased drastically during the 1980s. Someone finally decided it was appropriate for children with disabilities to participate in sports, as their able-bodied counterparts do. Whether it be the stipends provided to coaches of disabled sports programs within certain community school systems, the increasing number of summer sports camps for physically disabled children, or the specialized junior sports competitions being held throughout the United States, recent programming emphasis has begun to include our younger athletes.

Basic Opportunities

The United States Olympic Committee and most national governing bodies (NGB) have recognized for many years the importance of providing children with quality developmental programs. Many of the NGBs have developed extensive community-based sports programs for the younger athlete, while simultaneously fostering the growth of their future Olympic programs.

More importantly, in respect to children with disabilities, the discussion turns to a basic opportunity to participate. In most cases, involvement with a local disabled sport program represents the only opportunity for children with physical disabilities to participate in any type of organized athletics. The school systems that provide coaching stipends for interscholastic sports programs for students with physical disabilities are unfortunately the exception, not the rule. Although the implementation of PL 94-142 has increased the overall number of children with disabilities receiving adapted physical education over the past decade, a tremendous void still exists in overall programming.

The social, emotional, and physical benefits that able-bodied children receive from various intramural, interscholastic and community-sponsored sports programs are just as important for children with physical disabilities, if not more so.

Role of Physical Education

There is little doubt in my mind that physical education teachers are the unsung heroes behind today's superstars. Regardless of the sport, the initial interest, the basic motor patterns, and the physical skills that make the superstars what they are today are developed in the elementary and secondary physical education classes throughout the United States. This same result can and should be provided to children with physical disabilities. The slate of events offered by United States Cerebral Palsy Athletic Association (USCPAA) and the other Committee on Sports for the Disabled (COSD) groups can easily be incorporated into a physical education or adapted physical education curriculum (see Figure 1). A complete spectrum of physical education activities including individual, dual, team, and lifelong activities can be a part of a disabled student's program. Programs can also be established with both short- and long-term performance-based goals. Participation in local, regional, national, and even international competition provides an ideal goal-oriented format from which to structure a well-rounded curriculum. The diversity found within USCPAA also provides a number of ability-appropriate activities for students with cerebral palsy (CP) and les autres disabilities regardless of their functional capabilities.

Those athletes who feel they are not receiving adequate physical education instruction should encourage parents and coaches to begin educating teachers, therapists, and school administrators about the beneficial role they could be playing, not only in respect to the athletes' motor development and skill acquisition, but with their athletic achievements as well.

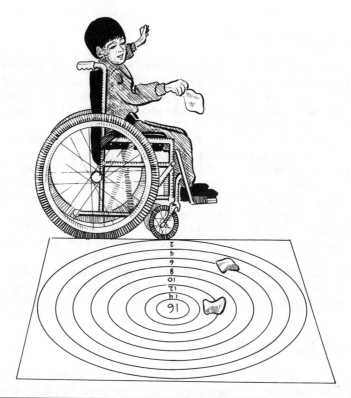

Figure 1.   The precision event as well as the other Class I field events can be easily incorporated into an adapted physical education curriculum.

Developing Effective Sports Programs

Age Appropriateness

A key part of providing sports programs for children is implementing age-appropriate activities. Similar to a properly structured physical education curriculum, a sports program involving children should meet the individual developmental needs of its participants. It is important for coaches to understand that at certain ages certain sports are very inappropriate and that within the sports that are appropriate, distances of events and size and weight of implements should be adapted to the particular age group.

An example of age appropriateness is outlined in Table 1, which lists the junior events offered by the Michigan Cerebral Palsy/Les Autres Sports Association. Events are introduced on a progressive manner within three age divisions leading developmentally to the events offered in the senior division category.

Adaptations in distances and implements are not the only changes made in Michigan's program when accommodating junior athletes. Competition organizers also take the time to instill a different type of competition philosophy when younger athletes are involved. Participation and fun are emphasized rather than winning

Table 1 Michigan CP/LA Sports Association, Youth Sports Events

Event	9 years and under	10–12 years	13–15 years
Track			
400/800 m	200-m fun run	200-m fun run	Same as Seniors
Field			
Shotput	Softball throw	Softball throw	4-lb shot only
Discus	Soft discus	Soft discus	Same as Seniors
Javelin	n/a	n/a	Same as Seniors
Long jump	Standing long jump	Standing long jump	Running long jump
Swimming	25 free and 25 back only	25 free and 25 back only	25 free and 25 back 50 free
Cycling			
Tricycle	400 m only	400 m only	800 m only
Bicycle	400 m only	800 m only	1500 m only
Powerlifting	n/a	n/a	13 to 14 years n/a 15 years only
Slalom	No ramp	No ramp	Same as Seniors

Note. Events not listed are offered without charge within each of three age categories. Boccia, archery, and target shooting are offered to Juniors within the Senior Division only. n/a = not available.

(Figure 2). Rules are more flexible, instruction is sometimes provided, and extra turns are given now and again.

Michigan's youth sports program has been in place since 1984 and has had alterations made each year since then. Changes are introduced based on input from coaches, competition organizers, and parents in hopes of continually providing the best programming possible. Again, the underlying concern is to appropriately meet the overall developmental needs of the children involved.

Cross-Disability Programs

Most programs providing activities for disabled youth are doing so through a cross-disability approach. This is because the majority of programs are being initiated by schools or community park and recreation departments. This type of programming allows children of various disabilities to participate together in all activities.

This trend is distinctly opposite from the disability specific disabled sports competitions held since the beginning of the disabled sports movement. Separate local, regional, national, and international competition is held annually for each of the seven COSD organizations, with few opportunities for combined or integrated competition.

Regardless of one's philosophical views concerning integrated and/or combined competition, one must agree with the decision of leaders within the field of youth sports to take the less complicated approach to competitions. Children with disabilities are different in enough ways without making them different among themselves. This cross-disability approach allows kids to be kids. If they stay involved in sports long enough to enter senior division competitions, they will be old enough to understand the need for different competitions.

Parents and the Little League Syndrome

One of the many similarities that can be drawn between organized sports programs for physically disabled youth and their able-bodied counterparts is a phenomenon

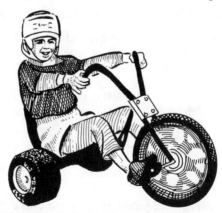

Figure 2.   A 9-year-old athlete with muscular dystrophy is allowed to ride a "Big Wheel" in the 400 m tricycle event.

I call "Little League Syndrome" (LLS). The causes of these physiological and psychological changes in parents of young competitors is very complex. What is clear is that the same pressures parents put on able-bodied children to succeed in sports are also placed on children with physical disabilities, and often more so.

Making a general analogy between parental involvement and a half-crazed mother or father in the bleachers of a Little League field is somewhat unfair and certainly not the intent of this chapter. Many programs, including several I have been involved with, depend extensively on and benefit greatly from the support provided by parents of the athletes. However, coaches of sports programs for children with disabilities will have to deal with parents as the Little League coach, basketball coach, and gymnastic instructor does. Yes, occasionally coaches will experience a parent suffering from LLS (see Figure 3).

More often though, parents of a disabled child will go through a cycle of expectations; from "no, my Johnny can't do that," to amazement over their child's seemingly impossible accomplishments; to finally, a "that's my boy" attitude. All of these reactions are very natural and to be expected. Coaches must understand that many of their athlete's parents have been blinded somewhat by the negativeness of diagnosis and long-term prognosis. Parents are not taught by doctors, therapists, or teachers to expect that their disabled child may be able to be successful in sports.

Once the parents have allowed their child to participate, coaches will be faced with those who want to get involved and those who do not. At times, involved parents can get biasedly overenthusiastic in respect to their own child's participation. A possible solution to this enthusiasm can be the creation of a team booster

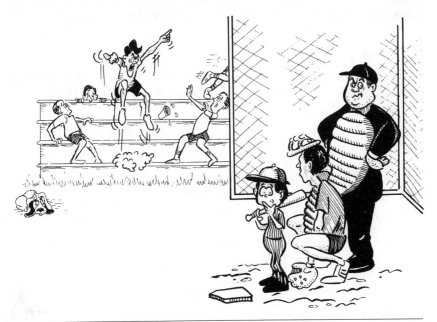

Figure 3. An occasional parent suffering from "Little League Syndrome" is to be expected.

club. Established to assist in team fund-raising, a booster club provides a goal to which parents' energies can be specifically channeled. Booster clubs allow parents to have a very meaningful role in the function of the team while at the same time allowing the coaching staff to attend to their responsibilities.

One final suggestion regarding parents is to educate those active in your program. Parents who are knowledgeable of rules and informed of current policies will be more likely to be an asset to your program.

Conclusion

Youth sports is the latest branch of programming to develop within the disabled sports movement. This chapter has attempted to outline several issues involved in providing services to younger athletes. It is strongly recommended that individuals interested in youth sports learn as much as possible about this newest group of participants to the competitive sports scene. One outstanding source of information is the Youth Sports Institute, 213 IM Sports Circle, Michigan State University, East Lansing, Michigan 48824, (517) 353-6689. Since 1979, the Youth Sports Institute has conducted more than 525 workshops involving more than 23,000 coaches. Workshop topics include program objectives, sports psychology, exercise physiology, growth and development, first aid, motor learning, discipline, parental involvement, and much more.

In respect to the child with CP, USCPAA has not yet developed a specific policy statement regarding youth sports (as of January, 1987). However, youth sports remains a key issue, demonstrated by the formation of a Youth Sports Subcommittee as part of the newly restructured National Sports Office (November, 1986).

Note

For more information on USCPAA's Youth Sports Program, contact: MaryBeth Jones, 31505 Kathryn, Garden City, MI 48135 or Carol Mushett, 34299 Claudia Court, Westland, MI 48185

Reference

Martens, R., Christina, R.W., Harvey, J.S., Jr., & Sharkey, B.J., (1981). *Coaching young athletes*. Champaign, IL: Human Kinetics.

Ingredients of Success

Gregory B. Shasby

Success is generally defined as the achievement of something desired, planned, or attempted. On an individual level the definition of success is relative to the specific goals one wishes to accomplish. For the most part, everyone will define success in a different way. Failure, however, has a universal definition. Failure is a person's inability to reach his or her goals in life, whatever they may be.

We all want to be successful. We all want to accomplish goals we have set for ourselves, but for some reason even the best planned attempts sometimes fall short. Why? Why are some people able to accomplish so much while others seem to flounder and never really achieve their desired goals?

The primary difference between those who have failed and those who have succeeded lies in the difference of their habits. It is estimated that at times 95% of our behavior is controlled by habits we have learned to perform automatically without having to think or decide. The learning and establishment of habits can, however, be either of a conscious or unconscious nature. Habits can be formed with a conscious awareness as to their function and role in directing behavior and therefore can be used to accomplish specific goals. On the other hand, habits can be formed as a function of highly emotional, random responses to the environment, resulting in primarily avoidance behavior. Although avoidance behavior may serve a protective function, more often it interferes with the ability to establish desired goals and more importantly to act in a way so as to accomplish the goals.

Because habit controls the majority of our behavior, success is dependent on the establishment of good habits. Consciously establishing good habits requires control principally over one thing, and that is your thoughts. You either control your mind or it controls you. All that you are is the result of what you have thought and currently think. The thoughts that you permit to predominate in your mind determine your character, your career, and your everyday life.

The key to success, then, is in controlling your thoughts. It rests with you to decide whether you are dominated by positive thoughts or negative thoughts. Two objects cannot fill the same space at the same time. The mind cannot be filled with negative thoughts or doubts if it is consciously and habitually filled with powerful and creative thoughts.

The most practical of all methods for controlling the mind is the habit of keeping it busy with a definite purpose or goal backed by a definite plan. The purpose or goal becomes the focal point for thought. The thoughts that predominate in your mind are associated with both the goal and the plan developed to accomplish the goal.

We need to establish goals in all areas of our lives. In establishing goals we want to establish habits of thinking that will enable us to utilize our talents, abilities, and interests to their fullest. We want to think creatively and think big, not limiting ourselves by preconceived notions of our abilities. The thinking that guides your intelligence and physical abilities is more important than how much intelligence and physical ability you have. Capacity is really a state of mind. How much we can do depends on how much we think we can do. No one accomplishes more than he or she sets out to accomplish. So, plan big. Set big goals. Let your dreams become your goals. Look to the top athletes in your class and let their performance levels become your goals.

A major stumbling block to successful goal setting is a lack of self-confidence. People who lack self-confidence are inwardly afraid and suffer from a deep sense of inadequacy and insecurity. Deep within themselves they mistrust their ability to meet responsibilities and grasp opportunities. They do not believe that they have it in them to be what they want to be. These fears and uncertainties lead to disorganization and lack of goal-directed behavior. Consequently, they make themselves content with something less than they are capable of.

The way to overcome these stumbling blocks is to create the right mental attitude through conditioned thought-habits. The attitude providing the basic structure to success in any venture is that of belief. Belief is essential in two areas. First, you must believe that the goal is obtainable, achievable, and within the realm of the possible. Second, you must believe in yourself and your ability to accomplish the desired goal. When you change your mental habits to belief instead of disbelief you learn to expect not to doubt. It is the act of believing that is the starting force or generating power that leads to accomplishment. Believe you can succeed and you will. Belief triggers the power to do. Through belief you bring everything into the realm of possibility.

Developing and maintaining a belief requires desire and affirmation. Desire is associated with the emotional aspects of experience. Desire is the emotion that is essential to the successful accomplishment of your personal goals. You must begin with desire if you ever hope to achieve anything. Nothing is as powerful as the desire to do something.

When desire becomes mixed with a faithful belief in yourself and a clearly defined goal, success is inevitable. The bond or interdependence between them is further strengthened by the quality of persistence. Persistence is the sustained effort necessary to accomplish the goal. Persistence provides the endurance necessary to carry you through the hard times. To get through those periods requiring extended effort and periods of wavering belief, persistence is the key.

The basis of persistence is the power of will, a positive state of mind. Because persistence is a state of mind, it can be cultivated. The steps leading to persistence include: (a) a definite purpose backed by a burning desire for its fulfillment; (b) a definite plan expressed in continuous action; (c) a mind closed tightly against all negative and discouraging influences, including negative suggestions by relatives, friends, and acquaintances; and (d) a friendly alliance with one or more persons who will encourage you to follow through with your plan.

Persistence requires energy, and energy is generated directly from the ingredients of success. When your mind is intensely interested in something you can keep at an activity indefinitely. You actually gain energy by losing yourself in something you strongly believe in and desire.

Closely tied to persistence is initiative. The best plans and the best intentions are of no use without action. Taking initiative, making decisions, and following through with plans is what completes the process. The secret of getting things done is to act.

One way to develop and maintain initiative is to make a habit of starting something new at least once a week. Another technique is to pair a key phrase with the action of beginning a task. Say the phrase, "Do it now" or "Go" before beginning a task. In the early stages of learning, never say the key phrase unless you follow through with desirable action. Start with little things and you will quickly develop the habit of a powerful reflex response.

Clearly defined goals, a strong desire to accomplish the goal, a belief in the goal and in yourself, and persistence are the ingredients of success. If used appropriately and wisely, they will ensure that you accomplish your goal with the least effort and greatest pleasure.

Appendix A
Directory of Sport and Recreation Organizations

Adapted Sports Association, Inc.
Communications Center
6832 Marlette Road
Marlette, MI 48453

Access Project
605 Eshleman
Berkeley, CA 94720

American Alliance for Health,
Physical Education, Recreation
and Dance
1900 Association Drive
Reston, VA 22091

American Association for Health,
Physical Education and Recreation
Programs for the Handicapped
1201 16th Street, N.W.
Washington, DC 20036

American Blind Bowling
Association
3500 Terry Drive
Norfolk, VA 23518

American Dance Therapy
Association
Suite 216E
1000 Century Plaza
Columbia, MD 21044

American Wheelchair Bowling
Association
15858 Larkspur Lane
Menominee Falls, WI 53051

American Wheelchair Pilots
Association
11018 102 Avenue North
Largo, FL 33540

The Amputee Golfers Association
Lakeview Terrace
Watchung, NJ 07060

Amputee Sports Association
P.O. Box 60129
Savannah, GA 31420-0129

American Athletic Association of the
Deaf
3916 Lantern Drive
Silver Spring, MD 20902
Richard Caswell
(301) 942-4042

Association for the Education of the
Visually Handicapped—Bulletin for
Physical Educators
919 Walnut Street
Philadelphia, PA 19103

The Association for the Severely
Handicapped (TASH), formerly
AAESPH
Garden View Suite
1600 W. Armory Way
Seattle, WA 98119

Berkeley Outreach Recreation
Program, Inc.
605 Eshleman Hall
University of California
Berkeley, CA 94720

Blind Outdoor Leisure
Development
533 East Main Street
Aspen, CO 81611

BOLD (Blind Outdoor Leisure
Development, Inc.)
513 Main Street
Aspen, CO 81611

Braille Sports Foundation
730 Hennepin Avenue, Room 301
Minneapolis, MN 55402

Canadian Association for Disabled
Skiing
Box 2077
Banff, Alberta
Canada, TO1 060

Canadian Wheelchair Sports
Association
333 River Road
Ottawa, Ontario, Canada K1L 889

California Wheelchair Aviators
Bill Blackwood, President
1117 Rising Hill
Escondido, CA 92025

Cerebral Palsy: International Sports
and Recreation Association
Dr. A. A. vanSchareven, Secretary
General
Heijneoordseweg 5
6813-GG Arhneim
The Netherlands

Disabled Sportsmen of America,
Inc.
P.O. Box 5496 (Hunting/Fishing)
Roanoke, VA 24021

Dwarf Athletic Association of
America
3725 West Holmes
Lansing, MI 48911

Goal Ball Championships
c/o Genie Kniebel
Butler University
Indianapolis, IN 46208

Handicapped Flyers International
1117 Rising Hill
Escondido, CA 92025

Handicapped Scuba Association
1104 El Prado
San Clemente, CA 92672

International Council on Therapeutic
Ice Skating
P. O. Box 13
State College, PA 16801

International Foundation for
Wheelchair Tennis
Peter Burwash, International
2203 Timberloch Place, Suite 126
The Woodlands, TX 77380

International Blind Sports
Organization
Bjorn Eklund, Secretary General
Shif Idrottens Hus
S-12387 Farstra, Sweden

International Coordinating
Committee of World Sports
Organizations for the Disabled
Heyenoordendeseweg 5
6813 GG Arhneim
The Netherlands

International Sports Organization for
the Disabled
Svensta Handikappidrotts
forbundet Idrottens Hus
S-12387 Farstra, Sweden

International Stoke-Mandeville
Games Federation
Sports Center for the Disabled
Harvey Road
Aylesburg, Bucks, England

International Wheelchair Road
Racers Club, Inc.
George Murray, President
Jeannette Parke, Secretary
165 78th Avenue, NE
St. Petersburg, FL 33702

National Beep Baseball Association
512 8th Avenue, NE
Minneapolis, MN 55413

National Consortium on Physical Education and Recreation for the Handicapped
Dr. John Hall, Membership Chairman
Physical Education Department
University of Kentucky
Lexington, KY 40506

National Foundation of Wheelchair Tennis
1544 Redhill Avenue, #A
Tustin, CA 92680

National Handicapped Sports and Recreation Association
Capitol Hill Station
P. O. Box 18664
Denver, CO 80218

National Inconvenienced Sportsman's Association
3788 Walnut Street
Carmichael, CA 95608

National Therapeutic Recreation Society
3101 Park Center Drive
Alexandria, VA 22302

National Wheelchair Athletic Association
2107 Templeton Gap Road, Suite C
Colorado Springs, CO 80907
(303) 632-0698

National Wheelchair Basketball Association
Stan Labanowich
110 Seaton Building
University of Kentucky
Lexington, KY 40506
(606) 257-1623

National Wheelchair Marathon
Bob Hall
15 Marlborough Street
Belmont, MA 02178

National Wheelchair Racquetball Association
c/o AARA

815 N. Weber, Suite 101
Colorado Springs, CO 80903

National Wheelchair Softball Association
Dave Van Buskirk, Commissioner
P.O. Box 737
Sioux Falls, SD 57101

North American Riding for the Handicapped Association
111 E. Wacker Drive
Chicago, IL 60601
(312) 644-6610

Ontario Wheelchair Sports Association
585 Tretheway Drive
Toronto, Ontario
Canada M6M 4B8

Ski for Light, Inc.
1455 W. Lake Street
Minneapolis, MN 55408
612-827-3232

Special Olympics
Suite 203
1701 K Street, N.W.
Washington, DC 20006

Sports for the Physically Disabled
333 River Road
Ottawa K1L 889 Canada

Tennis Association for the Mentally Retarded
22704 Ventura Boulevard, Suite 121
Woodland Hills, CA 91364

The 52 Association, Inc.
(Skiing-Blind, Amputee)
441 Lexington Avenue
New York, NY 10017
(212) 986-5281

United States Amputee Athletic Association
Richard Bryant
Bellforest Circle, Suite 149A
Nashville, TN 37221
(615) 662-2323

United States Association for
Blind Athletes
UAF/USC Benson Building
Gay Clement, ex-Director
Columbia, SC 29208
(803) 777-4465

United States Blind Golfer's
Association
c/o Patrick Browne Jr.
28th Floor
225 Baronne Street
New Orleans, LA 70112

United States Cerebral Palsy
Athletic Association
34578 Warren Road
Suite 264
Westland, MI 48184

United States Les Autres Sports
Association
c/o Dave Stephenson
5631 Alder, Apt. 7
Houston, TX 77081
(713) 664-9007

United States Deaf Skiers
Association
159 Davis Avenue
Hackensack, NJ 07601

United States Ski Association
Central Division
Amputee Skiers Committee
P.O. Box 66014
Chicago, IL 60666

Wheelchair Motorcycle Association,
Inc.
101 Torrey Street
Brockton, MA 02401

Wheelchair Pilots Association
11018 102nd Avenue, N.
Largo, FL 33540
(813) 393-3131

Wheelchair Sports Foundation
c/o Benjamin H. Lipton
40-24 62nd Street
Woodside, NY 11377

Additional Readings

American Academy of Orthopedic Surgeons. (1983). *Sports and recreational programs for the child and young adult with a physical disability.* Chicago: Author.

DePauw, K.P. (1984, February). Commitment and challenges: Sport opportunities for athletes with disabilities. *Journal of Physical Education, Recreation and Dance, 55*, 34–46.

United States Olympic Committee. (1982, August). *Handicapped in sports: A bibliography.* Colorado Springs, CO: USOC, Department of Education Services, Sports Medicine Division.

Appendix B
United States Cerebral Palsy Athletic Association

Sports Technical Committee

Committee Chairperson
Paul Tetreault
5 Beachwood Drive
N. Kingston, RI 02852

Chief Sports Technical Officer
Fred Koch
UCPA of New York City
175 Lawrence
Brooklyn, NY 11230

Boccia
Jamie McCole
1932 6th Avenue
Ft. Worth, TX 76110

Field Events
Rick Larder
5805 Woodward
Merriman, KS 66202

Bowling
Jerry McCole
Dallas Riders Disabled
   Sports Association
P.O. Box 3044
Dallas, TX 75221-3044

Powerlifting
Fred Koch
UCPA of New York City
175 Lawrence
Brooklyn, NY 11230

Cross-Country
George Brown
326 N. Quaker Lane
W. Hartford, CT 06119

Research
Claudine Sherrill
Texas Women's University
Denton, TX 76204

Cycling
Bob Accorsi
Recreation and Leisure Services
Springfield College
Springfield, MA 01109

Slalom Classification
Phil Kreuter
640 Ditmas Avenue, Apt. 10
Brooklyn, NY 11218

Equestrian
Mary Alice Goss
146 B-Kings Highway East
Atlantic Highland, NJ 07716

Soccer
Bernie Ruhlig
1770 Stillwell Avenue
Bronx, NY 10469

Swimming
Libby Anderson
1435 33rd Street
San Diego, CA 92102

Track
Paul Tetreault
5 Beechwood Drive
N. Kingston, RI 02852

Wheelchair Team Handball
Jeffery Jones
Michigan CP/LA Sports Association
P.O. Box 231
Garden City, MI 48135

Others

Athlete Representative to USOC
Duncan Wyeth
3147 Boston Boulevard
Lansing, MI 48910

USCPAA President
Grant Peacock, III
3132 Domar Forest Place
Decatur, GA 3033

Appendix C
Wheelchair Manufacturers

Blair Enterprises
6 Seco Court
Sacramento, CA
(916) 427-1035

Canadian Wheelchair
  Manufacturing, Ltd.
1312 Blundell Road
Mississauga, Ontario
Canada L4Y 1M5
(416) 275-3960

Everest & Jennings, Inc.
3233 East Mission Oaks Boulevard
Camarillo, CA 93010
(805) 987-6911

Hall's Wheels, Inc.
11 Smith Place
Cambridge, MA 02138
(617) 547-5000

Invacare, Inc.
899 Cleveland Street
P.O. Box 4028
Elyria, OH 44036
(216) 329-6000

Maraton Produkter
Adovagen
197 00 Bro
Sweden
0758-42540

XL Wheelchairs
4950-D Cohasset Stage Road
Chico, CA 95926
(916) 891-3535

Hand Crafted Metals, Inc.
13710 49th Street North
Clearwater, FL 33520
(813) 526-9416

Kuschall of America
15871 Edmund Drive
Los Gatos, CA 95030
(408) 438-6508

Shepherd Medical Products
P.O. Box 2249
Charlotte, NC 28211
(800) 833-9962

Competitive Engineering
5494 East Lamona Avenue, Suite 130
Fresno, CA 93727
(209) 251-4403

Magic In Motion, Inc.
239 West Stewart
Puyallup, WA 98371
(206) 848-6845

Magnum Poirier, Inc.
2930 West Central
Santa Ana, CA 92704
(714) 641-9696

Ortho-Kinetics, Inc.
W220 – N507 Springdale Road
P.O. Box 436
Waukesha, WI 52187
(414) 542-6060

Motion Designs, Inc.
2842 Business Park Avenue
Fresno, CA 93727
(209) 292-2171

CBS Cycle Frames Ltd.
1820 Trafalgar Street
Vancouver, British Columbia
Canada V6K 3S2
(604) 733-0758

Quadra Medical Products, Inc.
31166 Via Colinas
Westlake Village, CA 91362
(800) 824-1068

Sports Chairs
1673 Procyon Avenue
Las Vegas, NV 89103
(702) 873-6493

Stainless Medical Products
344 Airport Road
Festus, MO 63028
(800) 238-6678

E & G Sportschairs
2351 Parkwood Road
Snellville, GA 30278
(404) 972-0763,
(404) 972-0605

Wheel Ring, Inc.
175 Pine Street
Manchester, CT 06040
(203) 647-8596

Production Research Corp.
10217 Southard Drive
Beltaville, MD 20705
(301) 937-9633

Glossary

Scout Lee Gunn

Abduction. To draw away from midline of the body.

Acute. Sharp, severe; having rapid onset, severe symptoms and a short course; not chronic.

Adduction. To draw toward the midline of the body.

Ambulatory patient. The classification given to patients who are not confined to bed; usually patients in wheelchairs and on crutches are regarded as ambulatory patients.

Antagonist. A muscle acting in opposition to another.

Anatomical postures of the body. The terms used to describe anatomical postures are as follows:

Erect—body in a standing position.

Supine—body lying flat on the back in a horizontal position.

Prone—body lying face and trunk down in a horizontal position.

Laterally recumbent—body lying horizontally either on the right or left side.

Arthritis. A joint condition characterized by inflammation (redness), pain, swelling, and other changes varying with the type, common in the aging process. The general types of arthritis are:

Degenerative—You can think of this as the normal wear and tear upon joints and resulting in some disability and pain as you grow older. Occurs primarily in weight bearing joints, hips, and knees.

Rheumatoid—an actual disease process with the principal defect lying in the synovium, the fluid that lines and lubricates the joints. Because this is defective, the joints become involved and swelling, pain, and deformations result. This can affect any joint in the body, is chronic, and can begin in youth or during adulthood.

Arthrogryposis. A disease of the soft tissue and connective tissue that lies between the muscle cells resulting in multiple congenital contractures. Muscles are usually underdeveloped and are replaced by fibrous tissue and fat. The extreme fibrosis affects the joints resulting in the contractures. Most of these people are able to walk, but have very tight joints and are somewhat skinny. Again, the degree of involvement varies.

Ataxia. Lack of balance caused by muscular incoordination.

Atrophy. A wasting due to lack of nutrition or use of a part.

Body positions and directions. A number of anatomical terms are used in describing the body and determining position and direction. When the arms are hanging to the side, palms facing forward, with the body erect, the following terms are used to describe direction and position:

Anterior—toward the front or ventral side of the body.

Posterior—toward the back or dorsal side of the body.

Medial—nearer to or toward the midline.

Lateral—farther from the midline or the side of the body.

Internal—inside.

External—outside.

Pproximal—nearer to the point of origin or closer to the body.

Distal—away from the point of origin or away from the body.

Superior—above.

Inferior—below.

Cranial—toward the head.

Caudal—toward the lower end of the body (cauda means tail).

Cerebral palsy (CP). A disability due to damage of centers of the brain before or during birth resulting in imperfect control of the muscles and marked especially by muscular incoordination, spastic paralysis, and speech disturbances. It is estimated that more than half of the cerebral palsied are mentally retarded. The types of CP include

Spastic—characterized by jerky and uncertain movements and tightly contracting muscles.

Athetoid—typically showing uncontrolled, sprawling, muscular functioning.

Rigid—extremely tight muscles and limited, resistive movement.

Tremor—uncontrollably shaking limbs.

CVA. Cerebral vascular accident or stroke; caused by the following types of injury to the brain: blood clot, hemorrhage, compression, or trauma.

Chronic disabilities. Usually refers to those disabilities resulting from disease or conditions that may be slow-moving and progressive or in an arrested state, that is, where the progression or worsening has temporarily or permanently ceased.

Congenital. Existing at the time of or before birth.

Convulsion. A violent involuntary contraction of voluntary muscles, usually accompanied by loss of consciousness.

Cystic fibrosis A disease of the very young involving the endocrine glands, resulting in pancreatic insufficiency, chronic pulmonary disease, abnormally high sweat electrolyte levels, and sometimes cirrhosis of the liver; a fatal disease.

Dyslexia. Difficulty in reading; confusion of letters, "pot to top": defect in pathways that connect cerebellum (coordination) with the inner ear (balance).

Dystrophy. Defective nutrition or development.

Encephalitis. A general term used to delineate a diffuse inflammation of the brain. The condition may be acute or chronic and may be caused by a variety of agents such as viruses, bacteria, spirochetes, fungi, protozoa, and chemicals (such as lead). In addition to a number of neurological signs and symptoms, a variety of mental and behavioral changes occur during the illness and may persist beyond the acute phase of the illness.

Epilepsy. A disorder characterized by periodic motor or sensory seizures or their equivalents, and sometimes accompanied by a loss of consciousness or by certain equivalent manifestations. May be idiopathic (no known organic cause) or symptomatic (due to organic lesions). Usually accompanied by abnormal electrical discharge as shown by EEG.

Jacksonian epilepsy—recurrrent episodes of convulsive seizures or spasms localized in a part or region of the body without loss of consciousness. Named after Hughlings Jackson (1835–1911).

Major epilepsy—(grand mal): characterized by gross convulsive seizures with loss of consciousness.

Minor epilepsy—(petit mal): minor, nonconvulsive epileptic seizures or equivalents; may be limited to only momentary lapses of consciousness.

Psychomotor epilepsy—recurrent periodic disturbances, usually of behavior, during which the patient carries out movements often repetitive, highly organized but semiautomatic in character.

Extensors. Muscles that extend apart. A number of these muscles are in the wrists, fingers, ankles, and toes. See medical dictionary for proper names.

Flaccid. Limp, relaxed, and without muscle tone.

Flexors. Muscles that flex a joint. A number of these muscles are in the wrist, fingers, and foot. See medical dictionary for proper names.

Friedreich's ataxia. This is a fairly rare, progressive hereditary nervous disease beginning usually at about 8 to 12 years of age. It affects the parts of the spinal cord that mediate voluntary control, coordination, and postural sense and balance. Progression from walking with an unsteady walk to a wheelchair is the usual case. It may appear much like multiple sclerosis (MS) in the adult. Heart, diabetes and vision problems often occur in conjunction with the basic nervous condition.

Gait. Manner or style of walking.

Hydrocephalis. Increased accumulation of fluid in the protective layers of the brain, causing an enlarged head and face and disproportionately small eyes hidden in sockets and turned upward. May result from developmental anomalies, infection, injury, or brain tumors and is often accompanied by retardation.

Hyperactive. Excessive, above-the-normal use of energy or power of the mind.

Hypertonic. Abnormally great tension.

Hypertrophy. Abnormally large organ or part of the body, not due to a tumor.

Hypoactive. Slow, sluggish movement; less than usual use of energy or normal power of the mind. Apparent in the mentally retarded, brain injured, and emotionally disturbed.

Hypotonia. Diminished tension; reduction in muscle tone.

Incontinence. Loss of control of bladder or bowel or both.

Involuntary muscle. Muscle that cannot be moved at will.

Kinesthesia. The awareness of muscular motion, weight, and position.

Legg-Perthes disease. A diminished blood supply to the hip causing the bone to become shorter and the head of the thigh bone to become flat. Given time to heal by keeping weight off the hip usually corrects the problem, but this can take from 12 to 36 months.

Ligaments. Strong bands of tissue that hold bones together and keep organs in place.

Meningitis. Inflammation of the membranes surrounding the brain and spinal cord; can result in various types of brain damage.

Multiple sclerosis. There is an insulating layer of fatty substance over the brain and spinal cord, serving much like insulation over an electric wire and ensuring free passage of impulses; in the human, transmission of nervous impulses to the muscles. In multiple sclerosis (MS), this insulating layer for some reason breaks down; sclerotic patches occur in the brain and spinal cord and this interferes with the proper transmission of nervous impulses. The resultant course of this disease is one of ups and down, but usually progresses slowly downhill. Because of the damage to the nervous system, coordination, strength, speech, and/or eyesight may be compromised.

Muscular dystrophy (MD). There are several different types of muscular dystrophy, which is a genetic hereditary disease that results in a progressive wasting away of muscle.

Pseudohypertrophic—the wasted away muscle is replaced by fibrous tissue and fat. This type is transmitted from mother to son. The person may appear to have big muscular calves, buttocks, and shoulders. This disease affects primarily the trunk, shoulders, hips, calves, neck, and face muscles. Many die before they are 20 years old, not directly from MD but due to the lessening of respiratory functioning. The muscles controlling coughing are affected and thus mucous secretions stay in the lungs where it is warm and moist, creating a condition very conducive to infection and pneumonia. It is most important to guard against colds.

Amytonia congenita—(Oppenheim's disease)—a nonprogressive disorder in which there is a deficiency of the motor cells in the spinal cord that sends the message to the muscles. Because of this deficiency, the muscles are not fully innervated with the resultant weakness and lack of muscle tone. Because the person becomes older and bigger, he or she becomes even weaker, but the basic deficit does not get worse through it may appear to, due to body growth. As the person reaches full growth, the condition tends to stabilize. The same respiratory precautions as in MD should be followed in caring for these people.

Progressive spinal muscular atrophy—(Werdnig-Hoffman's disease)—the basic cause here is the same as in amytonia congenita, but here the nerve cells deteriorate and the disease is progressive, much like MD. This is also hereditary and begins during early childhood. It first affects the hips and thighs and later spreads to the extremities.

Perineal muscular atrophy—(Charcot-Marie Tooth disease)—a form of the above; also with hereditary tendencies and usually occurring in children. It involves progressive weakness of the distal muscles of the arms and feet near the ankles and hands.

Myotonia congenita—(Thompson's disease)—a rare inherited disease characterized by an excess of muscle tone, whereby the muscles are very rigid and unyielding with attacks of muscle spasm occurring.

Limb-girdle MD—involves progressive weakness and wasting of mainly the lower limbs, and usually begins after the age of 10.

Facial-scapular-humeral dystrophy—this type of dystrophy usually affects adults and involves the muscles of the face, shoulder blades, arms, and shoulders.

Nonambulant. A classification given to a patient unable to work or move about. A bed patient may be referred to as nonambulant.

Nonambulatory. Unable to walk independently, without assistance.

Orthopedics. Branch of medicine that deals with treatment of disorders involving locomotor structures of the body, especially the skeleton, joint, muscles, and fascia.

Parkinson's disease. A chronic nervous disease characterized by a fine, slowly spreading tremor, muscular weakness, and rigidity.

Pathology. Study of the nature and cause of disease that involves changes in structure and function.

Perceptual disorder. A cerebral impairment of the awareness of visual, auditory, or haptic stimuli.

Poliomyelitis (polio). Caused by a virus that affects the part of the spinal cord that sends out the motor message to the muscle. It does not affect the sensory part. The amount of degree of damage depends upon which parts of the spinal cord were affected, ranging from involvement of one leg to involvement of all extremities and the trunk. The muscles are thus deprived of their nerve output and waste away. Once the damage has occurred, it is nonreversible and yet nonprogressive.

Proprioception. Sensations arising from deeper body tissue such as muscles, ligaments, bones, tendons, and joints.

Prosthesis. Replacement of a missing part by an artificial substitute; an artificial organ or part.

Range of Motion (ROM). The extent of motion within a given joint. The types of ROM are:

Active—motion carried out voluntarily by the patient.

Active-Assistive—motion carried out voluntarily by the patient to the extent that it is possible for the patient with someone or something (such as a pulley) assisting him or her to complete the motion. (The patient has partial voluntary motion in the extremity).

Passive—motion is initiated and carried through by someone other than the patient or by the healthy part of the patient's body (e.g., a hemiplegic patient can use an unaffected arm to give passive ROM to the affected arm). The patient usually has little or no voluntary motion of the affected extremity.

Rigid. Constant resistance to movement. The spastic muscle will "give" and relax when it is moved to some degree, but rigidity means the muscles are generally very tight and stiff.

Scoliosis. A condition in which the spinal column is curved toward one side instead of normally straight. Severe cases can affect respiratory mechanism. Sometimes occurs in people with muscular dystrophy, or polio due to muscular imbalance in the back.

Shaping. Development of new behavior through systematic plans of reinforcement for successive approximations of the specific behavioral goal.

Spastic. Indicates there is an abnormal resistance to movement-tight muscles. This person will have a tendency to develop muscular contractures because of the brain lesion that interferes with free movement.

Spasticity. Hypertension of muscles causing stiff and awkward movements; the result of upper motor neuron lesion (damage to the brain cell).

Spasm. An involuntary, sudden movement or convulsive muscular contraction.

Spina bifida. "Bifid" means short, thus a "short spine." This is a congenital malformation of the spinal cord and the supporting vertebral column causing the spinal cord to herniate through causing paralysis below this point. Most of the time this occurs in the low back and the person will have a surgical scar and/or remnants of the "bif." Most people usually have some use of their upper legs and are able to walk with crutches and/or braces. The nerves to the bowel and bladder are always impaired and the person may have a type of urinary receptacle, use suppositories, or be on a regular time schedule for bowel movements. Many have slightly enlarged heads due to the trauma to the spinal cord, upsetting the balance of spinal fluid and causing an increase of pressure in the head. This is known as hydrocephalus and also occurs apart from spina bifida. The spinal cord and brain are bathed in spinal fluid, which is produced and reabsorbed into the bloodstream in the brain. This fluid circulates up and down, bathing the brain and the spinal cord. Due to congenital or developmental defects in this system, blockage of channels, and so on, an increase of pressure and a resultant increase in skull size occurs. This can cause neurological and mental damage and the degree of damage will again vary a great deal.

Tonus. State of tension, present to a degree in muscles at all times.

Reference

All terms and definitions were taken from:

Gunn, S.L. (1975). *Basic terminology for therapeutic recreation and other action therapies* (pp. 21–22, 24–25, 27–34, 40, 42–43, 49–54). Champaign, IL: Stipes. (4th printing)